C000157980

The
Economics
of *Therapy*

Caring for Clients,
Colleagues, Commissioners and
Cash-Flow in the Creative Art Therapies

Edited by Daniel Thomas and Vicky Abad
Foreword by Brynjulf Stige

Jessica Kingsley *Publishers*
London and Philadelphia

First published in 2017
by Jessica Kingsley Publishers
73 Collier Street
London N1 9BE, UK
and
400 Market Street, Suite 400
Philadelphia, PA 19106, USA

www.jkp.com

Copyright © Jessica Kingsley Publishers 2017
Foreword copyright © Brynjulf Stige 2017

Library of Congress Cataloging in Publication Data
Title: The economics of therapy / edited by Daniel Thomas and Vicky Abad.
Description: London ; Philadelphia : Jessica Kingsley Publishers, 2017. |
    Includes bibliographical references and index.
Identifiers: LCCN 2016050379 (print) | LCCN 2016053875 (ebook) | ISBN
    9781849056281 (alk. paper) | ISBN 9781784502195 (ebook)
Subjects: | MESH: Sensory Art Therapies--economics | Practice
    Management--economics | Models, Organizational
Classification: LCC RC489.A72 (print) | LCC RC489.A72 (ebook) | NLM WB 555 |
    DDC 615.8/5156068--dc23

British Library Cataloguing in Publication Data
A CIP catalogue record for this book is available from the British Library

ISBN 978 1 84905 628 1
eISBN 978 1 78450 219 5

Printed in Great Britain

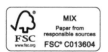

Dedication

Daniel Thomas

To Wendy, Daisy and Florence love-dee love-dee love-dee, from Daddy xxx.

Vicky Abad

To Jose and Arwen, you are the inspiration behind the business, you are my everything.

Contents

Foreword
Phases of transition in the economics and ethics of the arts therapies
Brynjulf Stige

Funding therapy is a practical concern, but it is also much more than that. The financial side of therapeutic practice also calls for philosophical reflection; it involves values-based choices in relation to issues such as fair access, service quality, and reasonable compensation. For these reasons, I would argue that the arts therapists would benefit from relating to economics as a social science, alongside other social sciences of relevance, such as anthropology and sociology. As a social science, economics is concerned with factors that govern the production, consumption, and distribution of goods and services. Equality and solidarity are among the values that many arts therapists cherish, which suggests that the distribution aspect of economics is key for our professions.

According to a number of economists, the dynamics of capitalism, the dominating economic system around the world today, creates structures of unjust inequality (Piketty 2014). This hardly comes as a surprise to anyone who pays attention to the developments in the world we live in. While there was considerable optimism in the decades after World War II about the possibility of modifying capitalism in the service of more equality, inequities have again been raising dramatically since the 1970s and 1980s. The neo-liberalism supported by politicians such as Thatcher and Reagan has been a driving force, and in some countries today, inequality is so extreme that discontent generates considerable challenges to democratic values and practices. The global financial crisis that began in 2008 has accentuated the appraisal that we are dealing with a failing system, and some economists have started to ask how capitalism will end

(Streeck 2016). Arts therapists might think that it is beyond their area of competence to contribute with answers to such a question. I would argue that it is important that we do at least consider the strengths and weaknesses of a capitalist system.

Obviously, inequality in health is an area of concern, and it might be helpful to distinguish between inequality and inequity. Used as a descriptive term, inequality denotes differences, for instance in biological disposition for diseases. *Inequity* refers to avoidable differences. Consequently, inequities are unfair and unjust. When we describe global differences in health problems, medical language might be helpful for specification of diseases and disorders, while various therapy discourses might enhance our understanding of people's experiences. Neither of these discourses depict very well the social and economic mechanisms involved, however. The disciplines of sociology and economics provide us with a much better understanding of the conditions and processes that create health inequities (Stige & Aarø 2012, pp.59–87). For instance, Wilkinson and Pickett (2010) have documented that pronounced socioeconomic differences produce health inequities. Perhaps more surprising, they also found that such differences lead to increased health challenges for all groups in society, not only for disadvantaged groups. The main explanation is that socioeconomic differences are associated with less social cohesion, whereas we need increased social cohesion for better health. This is an appraisal we also know from Putnam's (2000) influential study of social capital. We cannot afford the rich (Sayer 2015), and this seems to be the case in health economics as well.

With this book, we finally have a publication that addresses the financial side of practicing therapy, including, but going beyond, the business of doing business. The book does include several chapters about how to grow and sustain a business but in addition, many chapters include discussions about ethics (Chapter 5), the value of therapy (Chapter 4), and problems of structural violence (Chapter 7), to name a few of the themes emerging from a range of national and cultural contexts.

One argument made in the book is that the global financial crisis in 2008 makes it more relevant for therapists to own their own therapy businesses, so that they can develop high quality services and be less dependent on government funding, which arguably has been unstable in many countries. My appraisal is that the global financial crisis makes it more crucial than ever to work for strengthened government funding of the arts therapies, because government involvement is key in the process of countering inequities in health. Perhaps this difference in appraisal mainly reflects differences in focus, but the economics of the arts therapies could not and should not be a unified field. The chapters of this book demonstrate that a number of perspectives inform the emerging discourse. Some differences might relate to the diverse social, cultural, and economic contexts that shape our work, others might reflect disparities in values and priorities. Other differences again reflect various levels of analysis: What could each therapist do, and what is ethical in relation to each patient or participant? What could our associations and organisations do, and what is ethical in relation to society as a whole?

'There is no such thing as society,' Margaret Thatcher famously claimed in the 1980s, a statement which could stand as an epitaph for the values of the neoliberal era emerging at the time. As a social science, mainstream economics has largely reflected the ethos of individualist cultures (Hofstede, Hofstede & Minkov 2010, pp.128–129). When the discipline was founded in 18th century Britain, Adam Smith was one of the founding fathers. His influential economic theory was based on the assumption that each individual's pursuit of self-interest in a market increases the wealth of nations. The fact that Smith distinguished between self-interest and selfishness and that he had developed a theory of moral sentiments as well, stressing the 'fellow feeling' of sympathy as particularly important, is often ignored. In any case, mainstream economic theory is based on the image of the individual, rational actor, so that there has been a tendency to downplay the social nature and the history of humankind (Torsvik 2003). It is perhaps beyond the mandate and competencies of arts therapists to redress the theoretical limitations of the discipline of economics, but in our dealings with economics we cannot overlook them. This is particularly critical in phases of transition; phases when the macroeconomics of society change, with implications for the microeconomics of the arts therapies. The aftermath of the global financial crisis in 2008 could be seen in this light.

Phases of transition also emerge because cultural and political changes at the macro level induce changes in the funding of services, sometimes with possibilities for creating new posts, sometimes not. My own experiences with such phases include working with the creation of government-funded music therapy positions within the 'economics of inclusion' that emerged in Norway in the 1980s (Kleive & Stige 1988), and within the 'economics of empowerment' that characterises the current turn to recovery-oriented practice within services for people with mental health and substance use challenges (Stige 2016). Of course, any therapist's work with the funding of services is grounded in macroeconomics. My own work is based in the Nordic model of social democracy, which attempts to combine a capitalist system with regulations and political actions that promote social justice (Moene & Wallerstein 2001). Work grounded in political systems with less emphasis on redistribution and universal access to healthcare will necessarily be different, and it is therefore highly pertinent that this book includes chapters from a number of countries and cultures. As several of the chapters exemplify, no system or economic trend is inevitable; they are maintained by people's practices.

Therapeutic activities affect, and are affected by, economic and social structures, and even though many traditions of therapy have focused on individual change, I would argue that any tendency of describing the world in terms of dualisms between the individual and the society should be challenged (Stige 2015). Therefore, the economics of the arts therapies not only concerns the quality of services and the financial security of the therapists, but the realisation of the rights of service users as well. Several decades ago, Even Ruud (1980) argued that music therapy services have limited meaning if we ignore socioeconomic conditions. This theme has been developed lately, in relation to how we understand people's problems (Helle-Valla 2016) and how we think about the sustainability of our activities (Bolger & Skewes McFerran 2013).

Our individual powers to change the world are limited, but through various partnerships, change might be within reach (Stige & Aarø 2012). In Chapter 2 of this book, Alison Ledger makes a case for *entrepreneurship* in the arts therapies. She endorses a broad definition of the term by referring to innovative involvement with the uncertainties and complexities of the world. Consequently, she also refers to a shift in interest from the individual entrepreneur to social *processes* of entrepreneurship. Ledger's (2016) previous work on the creation of music therapy posts has demonstrated that many music therapists feel isolated and insecure when developing services. Her interest in processes of entrepreneurship is highly pertinent, then, and I would argue that collaborative processes of entrepreneurship should be given much more attention in our professions. Our associations, universities, and organisations all have roles to play in such processes (Stige 2016).

Again, the relevance of the argument relates to phases of transition. For instance, when national treatment guidelines in several countries have started to recommend consideration of the arts therapies (e.g. NICE 2013; The Norwegian Directorate of Health 2013), the possibilities and responsibilities of our professions change. We obviously have to consider the quality of our services, but the context of considering the quantity and identity of services has changed as well. Recommendations like these have little value if the available numbers of arts therapists are so low that services in practical terms would be available only to a few, even if funding were available. Also, as Edwards (2015) and others have suggested, with statutory recognition comes regulation. Such a phase of transition substantially influences issues of professional identity, then. Some music therapy researchers, for instance, have expressed concerns about the risk of adjusting our practices too much to a medical model, while service users often highlight the value of the non-medical nature of these practices, even to the degree of suggesting that music therapy is the opposite of treatment (Solli & Rolvsjord 2015).

As this book makes perfectly clear, the economics of therapy can not be separated from the ethics of practice. The argument I have indicated above is that ethics goes beyond the issue of not doing harm at the individual level to include issues such as solidarity and social justice (Stige 2012). The economics of the arts therapies, therefore, is the basis for a number of crucial questions about research, theory, and practice. Which questions do we ask? How do we understand human problems and possibilities? Which people and places do we serve, and how? Economics is key to the funding of what we already do or want to do, but also to continued development of the role and the identity of the arts therapies in society. Not all of these questions are addressed in this book, of course, but the various chapters contribute substantially to the discourse on the economics of therapy.

References

Bolger, L., and Skewes McFerran, K. (2013). Demonstrating sustainability in the practices of music therapists: Reflections from Bangladesh. *Voices: A World Forum for Music Therapy*, 13, 2. doi:10.15845/voices.v13i2.715.

Edwards, J. (2015). Paths of professional development in music therapy: Training, professional identity and practice. *Approaches: Music Therapy & Special Music Education*, 7, 1, 44-53.

Helle-Valle, A. (2016). How do we understand children's restlessness? A cooperative and reflexive exploration of children's restlessness as a bioecological phenomenon. Unpublished doctoral dissertation, The Grieg Academy, University of Bergen.

Hofstede, G., Hofstede, G.J. and Minkov, M. (2010). *Cultures and Organizations: Software of the Mind: Intercultural Cooperation and Its Importance for Survival*. New York: McGraw Hill.

Kleive, M. and Stige, B. (1988). *Med lengting, liv og song. Prøveordning med musikktilbod for funksjonshemma i Sogn og Fjordane* [With Longing, Life, and Song: Music for People with Disabilities in The County of Sogn og Fjordane] Oslo: Samlaget.

Ledger, A. (2016). Developing New Posts in Music Therapy. In J. Edwards (ed.) *Oxford Handbook of Music Therapy*. Oxford: Oxford University Press.

Moene, K. and Wallerstein, M. (2001). Inequality, social insurance, and redistribution. *American Political Science Review*, 95, 4, 859-874.

NICE (2013). *Psychosis and schizophrenia in children and young people: Recognition and management*. London: National Institute for Health and Clinical Excellence; NICE clinical guideline 155. Retrieved from https://www.nice.org.uk/guidance/cg155 on 1 December 2016.

Piketty, T. (2014). *Capital in the Twenty-First Century* [translated by Arthur Goldhammer]. Cambridge, MA: Belknap Press.

Putnam, R. (2000). *Bowling Alone: The Collapse and Revival of American Community*. New York: Simon and Schuster.

Ruud, E, (1980). *Hva er musikkterapi?* [What is Music Therapy?]. Oslo: Gyldendal Norsk Forlag.

Sayer, A. (2015). *Why We Can't Afford the Rich*. Bristol: Policy Press.

Solli, H.P. and Rolvsjord, R. (2015). 'The opposite of treatment': A qualitative study of how patients diagnosed with psychosis experience music therapy. *Nordic Journal of Music Therapy*, 24, 1, 67-92, doi: 10.1080/08098131.2014.890639.

Stige, B. (2012). *Elaborations Toward a Notion of Community Music Therapy* (ebook, revised edition). Gilsum, NH: Barcelona Publishers.

Stige, B. (2015). The practice turn in music therapy theory. *Music Therapy Perspectives*, 3, 1, 3-11, doi: 10.1093/mtp/miu050.

Stige, B. (2016). *Creating posts for music therapists within the changing realities of contemporary health care systems – how is that related to theory, research, and ethics?* Keynote at the 10th European Music Therapy Conference, Vienna, 05–09 July, 2016.

Stige, B. and Aarø, L. E. (2012). *Invitation to Community Music Therapy*. New York: Routledge.

Streeck, W. (2016). *How Will Capitalism End? Essays on a Failing System*. London: Verso.

The Norwegian Directorate of Health (2013). Utredning, behandling og oppfølging av personer med psykoselidelser (IS 1957) [Assessment, Treatment, and Follow-up of Persons with Psychotic Disorders]. Oslo: The Norwegian Directorate of Health.

Torsvik, G. (2003). *Menneskenatur og samfunnsstruktur: Ein kritisk introduksjon til økonomisk teori* [Human Nature and Social Structure: A Critical Introduction to Economic Theory]. Oslo: Samlaget.

Wilkinson, R. and Pickett, K. (2010). *The Spirit Level: Why Equality Is Better for Everyone.* London: Penguin.

Acknowledgements

Writing a book such as this, which we hope breaks new ground, is wonderfully challenging and also difficult. Our primary acknowledgements are for our chapter writers who have contributed their ideas, energy, experience, questions and queries in the most generous of ways – without them this book would have remained a few sentences on the back of an envelope.

We also would like to thank colleagues in Chroma and Boppin' Babies. At Chroma we thank Wendy Thomas, Andrew Bailey, Jo Godsal, Kate Cropper, Liz Turley and Jenny Jenkins. At Boppin' Babies we thank the leadership team: Jose Abad, Kate Fletcher, Chare Walton, Emily Diamond and Sheryl Davies. We thank you all for your support, understanding and interest in thinking about and developing sustainable business models for therapy services. A warm debt of gratitude goes to Martin Davies for his patient and generous mentoring which has contributed hugely to Chroma's growth and how we think about the business, and to Emily Diamond for her mentoring and guidance as we bopped along and grew at Boppin' Babies.

Thanks go to family members who support us to run our businesses and write books, including Sheryl, Jose, David, Stevie, Elizabeth, Sian and Pete, and because you are the people who tell us we can do it and keep us going with your optimism and spirit.

Finally a big thank you to all the music, art and drama therapists in Chroma and the registered music therapists and music teachers in Boppin' Babies for their tireless and wonderful work out there in the world, which is always where the value of our work is most accurately measured.

Daniel & Vicky, February 2017

Introduction
Daniel Thomas and Vicky Abad

Economics and therapy. Therapy and economics. Two unlikely bedfellows? While economics and therapy may seem poles apart, current cross-discipline research, ideas and thinking (Pink 2014), and the day-to-day experience of therapy business owners across the world, suggest otherwise. The fact is that without economics, we can't have therapy. Without funding we can offer nothing. These are the facts. Once we accept this, the focus moves to where the funding comes from, and how sustainable current funding models are.

The financial health of creative arts therapists, both individually and as a profession, has the potential to impact the work we do and therefore the health and well-being of our clients. Our profession sits within large and often financially constrained health, education and social care ecosystems. Without financial health, therapists, therapy businesses and professional organisations cannot provide the clinical work that is paramount to the greater health and well-being of our clients and our communities. Can we care for our clients, colleagues, commissioners and cash-flow in a healthy, self-sustaining way, while staying aligned with our Code of Ethics to do no harm?

This book addresses this question by exploring two key economic issues: our attitudes towards operating for-profit therapy businesses, and transferring the skills that we already possess as highly trained therapists to the business world. Therapists possess core therapeutic and clinical skills, honed over many years of training and through use every single day in practice, which can and should be transferred to develop and grow high quality, profitable and sustainable therapy services.

Terminology

Throughout this book, we use the terms 'arts therapist' and 'creative arts therapist/therapy' as a way to describe a broad range of professionals and professions. These include:

- art therapy/art psychotherapy
- drama therapy
- music therapy
- dance and movement therapy
- play therapy.

While relevant to a wide range of people, this book has been written with therapeutic practitioners in mind. We hope the ideas shared over the following 11 chapters will be of interest to creative arts therapists, psychotherapists, occupational therapists, speech and language therapists, counsellors and trainee therapists, regardless of whether they work in private practice, are employed or are on professional placements.

Within this book, we use of the term 'commissioner' to refer to anyone who purchases therapy services on behalf of a client group or individual. This may include school leaders, hospital managers, social workers, parents and other professionals.

Context of the book

This book was conceived during the Global Financial Crisis (GFC) of 2008 and its subsequent impact on traditional funding models. We believe that many of the funding model changes that occurred as a consequence of the GFC are here to stay. In many areas of the world, the GFC still continues eight years later. Financial cycles of good times and hard times seem to be a part of what all businesses, workers and self-employed therapists have to manage and overcome. It's often easier in the good times, however, to ignore the need to build the robust business structures to survive the hard times. Regardless of where the world economy is when you read this book, we hope our ideas cultivate discussion and a new awareness of the issues raised.

Aim of the book

This book first aims to challenge therapists to think about funding and money in a more empowered way. It aims to reframe our ideas of funding and to support therapists in adopting self-sufficiency when thinking about money, rather than relying on governments to fund their work. Second, this book aims to empower therapists to recognise the skills they already possess and use these to build their business practice. We believe there are core therapy skills that we possess through innate ability and tertiary training that meet both therapeutic and business needs alike.

Structure of the book

This book is structured into three broad areas:

Part 1 encompasses the first two chapters and sets the scene for the book – what does funding look like in the 21st century and what do commissioners want? In Chapter 1 we provide an overview and reflection of the financial changes experienced so far this century and examine the potential impact these have on arts therapies funding. We then examine more deeply what funding bodies are actually looking for. How do we meet these needs in the face of changing funding structures? Alison Ledger explores some of these issues in Chapter 2, including service development.

Part 2 begins with Chapter 3, where we look more closely at the 'how' – how do we meet the needs of commissioners and funding bodies in an ever-reducing funding climate? What skills do we already possess that we can tap into? We present core skills we believe therapists possess that go a long way to meeting these needs, skills we are already highly trained in. In Chapter 4, Monika Geretsegger, Elena Fitzthum and Thomas Stegemann delve more deeply into the dilemmas therapists face when determining the value of therapy, such as setting fees and asking for money. While this is something we all need to do if we want to eat, some people are more comfortable accepting money indirectly through employment than they are through charging directly for their services. This leads us to ethics – how do we charge and work in a private practice model in an ethical and transparent way? Stine Jacobsen shares her knowledge and ideas on this in Chapter 5.

We believe all therapists would be more adept at charging for their work if tertiary/professional training included guidelines and examples of how to run successful businesses and organisations, even if this means thinking about how to become 'just' self-employed.

Part 3 starts with Chapter 6. In this chapter, Petra Kern provides a detailed example of how she teaches students about therapy and business skills in her tertiary training programme. In Chapter 7 Rebecca Zarate provides an American perspective on business in the creative arts therapies, before we look at how clinicians have set up for-profit creative arts therapy businesses in different parts of the world.

Chapters 8 to 11 share four case studies from four different countries. The first case study, in Chapter 8, is written by Elaine Matthews Venter, an arts therapist based in Auckland, New Zealand, who provides practical and user-friendly information and examples on how she set up a new clinical area of practice in her country. She provides many easy-to-use take-home messages and ideas throughout. Chapter 9 provides an example of a business that started small and grew up. Advantages and disadvantages to this business model are shared in an open and frank way by Vicky Abad. Chapter 10 provides a case study that is quite the opposite – Daniel Thomas shares how he started with a big idea and is continually building his business towards that vision. Chapter 11 provides an interesting and unique look at how Kingman Chung set up his business in Asia to meet market demand within the context of a complete lack of government funding or funded positions in his country. His story is truly inspiring.

We hope you enjoy the book and find it useful.

Background to the text

This book has evolved out of conversations between two colleagues who became friends. Conversations followed over coffee, face-to-face and jetlagged in airports, on Skype and on Facebook, about the different business models we were using and the successes and failures of each. We began to see commonalities that we believed were the underpinnings of our growing businesses despite quite different business models, clinical practices and populations. We also noticed these common traits existed despite the very real economic downturn the world was experiencing at the time. In light of the impact on funding trends, we began to think about two seemingly different yet interrelated things – how to change the way people think about funding and our financial health as a professional group, *and* how to help colleagues tap into their own clinical strengths to work more effectively outside of traditional funding models.

More conversations followed, books and resources were shared, and we began to pull together a model for a therapy business that looked nothing like anything we had seen in that space. We wanted to find a way to share this with our colleagues – to say to them, 'You are great! You can do this – and here's how.' We presented our business model at the 39th Australian Music Therapy Conference in Melbourne in 2013 and really got tongues wagging. We heard from colleagues who really liked what we had to say and the way our thoughts were heading, and we pulled together a round table for the 14th World Congress of Music Therapy in Krems, 2014.

This book is the culmination and continuing working collaborations of that round table, and the ever-developing business models and minds of Daniel and Vicky. It is all about making sense of the things we are really good at – the core clinical strengths we have developed over many years of training and practice that we feel apply equally to business, and understanding the systems well enough to make a go of it. And it is about collaborating with each other, with our colleagues, with our clients and our communities to create businesses that can look after them as well as cash-flow and commissioners in caring and ethical ways.

Reference
Pink, D. (2014). *To Sell is Human*. Edinburgh: Canongate Books Ltd.

CHAPTER 1

The Economics of Therapy
Caring for Clients, Colleagues, Commissioners and Cash-flow
Daniel Thomas and Vicky Abad

Introduction

How are economics and therapy alike? What commonalities do they share? We know participation in the arts is good for our health, and in some cases even saves money. We know healthy people cost society less. We also know therapy costs money. And finally, from our experience as therapists and therapy service developers, we also know that business and therapy share a common core – relationships. Relationships are built between consumers and products, consumers and manufacturers, consumers and sales staff, and between therapists and clients, therapists and school leaders, therapists and colleagues. So let's begin with a strengths-based approach, to see what we are very good at doing as therapists, and how this relates to business.

Recent literature reviews suggest that engagement with the arts can have significantly positive effects on health (Chlan 1998; Davies *et al.* 2012; Davies, Knuiman & Rosenberg 2016; Stuckey & Nobel 2010). Within the arts therapy professions, studies highlight specific areas such as the common belief that music participation and music listening are 'innately good' (Edwards 2011, p.90). More specifically, music's ability to calm neural networks (Krout 2006) and its capacity to reduce stress and anxiety are widely recognised (Guzzetta 1989). Staricoff (2006) found that art therapy patients were significantly more likely to have improved clinical outcomes, including better vital signs, diminished cortisol related to stress, and less medication needed to induce sleep than those who did not participate in any arts therapies. Within expressive writing, dance and movement therapy and dramatherapy, results showed significant quality-of-life improvements within the intervention groups. In 2005, Sandel and colleagues conducted pilot research at two cancer centres in Connecticut to determine the effects of a dance and movement programme on quality of life, shoulder function, and body image among breast cancer survivors treated within the preceding five years. Within the intervention group, shoulder range of motion and body image increased at 13 weeks. This pilot programme substantially enhanced quality-of-life indicators for study participants by addressing their post-treatment physical and emotional needs (Sandel *et al.* 2005).

Across the general population the creative arts therapies are used within a spectrum of prevention, early intervention and treatment settings. Through their specialised training and person-centred care and treatment pathways, art, drama and music therapists are well positioned to provide clients with a range of health benefits. Bruscia's (1998) use of 'ecological' to contextualise music therapy practice that goes beyond traditional frameworks of client, therapist and confidentiality is helpful when trying to think about music (and other therapies) in the 21st century. 'Ecological' suggests a potentially sustaining and 'naturally healthy' series of relationships that self-regulate, evolve and support diversity.

Bruscia's use of the term seeds ideas of wellness and harmony, and may also reflect back a time when everything was wholesome and undisturbed. However, all systems, regardless of type, require inputs and outputs to find an equilibrium that creates an overall healthy balance. Within the creative arts therapy ecological system, therapists have traditionally focused on outputs to clients and patients, but are less sure-footed when thinking about the financial health and well-being inputs of therapy business, organisation or single-therapist practices. Therapy does not exist in a vacuum, and although many of us find our work hugely satisfying and stimulating, we cannot work for free – we have mortgages, holidays, childcare, food and expenses to pay for. Funding to provide the necessary services to meet these health outcomes is inconsistent and variable across region and country. This is despite the fact that our professions are well positioned to provide a range of evidence-based health benefits and that we are constantly gaining greater recognition for our ability to deliver positive health outcomes.

We hope this chapter is the starting point of a new way of conceptualising how creative arts therapists think about their work from inside and outside the therapy space. Using therapeutic ideas of containment and boundaries, we can think of the relationship between 'sessional content' (the client, the therapist, the process of therapy, etc.) and the 'operating context' (strategic government policy, commissioning, funding, evaluation, ethics, etc.) as the yolk/white and shell of an egg respectively. The shell (operating context) needs to be robust, strong and transparent enough to protect, warm and nurture what it contains; the yolk/white (sessional content) needs to be nutritious, alive and safe from outer disturbances and influences. Both the shell and the yolk/white are required for growth and development. Within therapy, these two elements support the client to evolve and develop increasingly independent mental, physical, social, societal and spiritual ways of being.

Background to a new way of thinking

From 2008 onwards, gross domestic product (GDP) fell across many Western countries for consecutive years, including the two countries we live in – the UK (Daniel) and Australia (Vicky). Central government spending cutbacks in core social service provision continued to be implemented, while evidence linking economic disadvantage to lower educational attainment, shortened life expectancy, social and family breakdown and compromised health outcomes grew. Traditional funding sources for a range of therapy services dropped off the cliff as cutbacks bit hard into departmental budgets. In the UK, demand for mental health services rose by a staggering 20 per cent from 2008 to 2013 while mental health service budgets were cut by 8 per cent in real terms (McNicoll 2015).

Europe and North America were particularly hard hit by the Global Financial Crisis (GFC). In the UK, the National Council for Voluntary Organisations (NCVO 2013) predicted that charities would lose £2.8 billion in public funding between 2011 and 2016. Other countries experienced near total economic collapse in their banking systems and social welfare models, and some continue to report very high unemployment levels in 2016 (Tadeo & Duarte 2016). While there is economic recovery through small-scale 'green-shoots' growth, the reality is fewer people are doing the work of many, and more people are relying on charity for survival. The *New York Times* reported that American food banks provided assistance to more than 37 million Americans in 2012 through more than 61,000 outlets (Korkki 2012).

In Australia the effects of the GFC were softened by an economic stimulus package instigated by the Rudd Labour government. Australia was not entirely immune – Queensland Health, for example, suffered severe funding cuts of at least AUD $103 million between 2012 and 2015, leading to nearly 3000 healthcare job losses. Other non-health government sectors have been equally hard hit. In Victoria, the Eastern Health sector saw all of the music therapy positions cut, and other health departments reported feelings of threat. In the aftermath of the financial crisis, many economists predicted that the old models were out; governments would not have the money to fund future health and community care in the same way or to the same degree as they used to.

Within any financial funding context, the role of the therapy business is to provide an operating context (the shell) that creates a potential space (Winnicott 1973), within which the therapy can take place and develop according to the needs of each client. Just as the baby and mother are indivisibly linked within the process of play and child development, so too are the sessional content (the yolk/white) and the operating context (the shell) within the economics of therapy.

How is therapy funded?

Traditionally, many creative arts therapists are either employed by governments, or work in not-for-profit, statutory or charitable sectors that are funded directly or indirectly by governments. Are we, as professionals, comfortable to sit within this 'dependency' funding model? There are of course exceptions, and this can be seen most notably in the United States, where therapists owning therapy businesses are more commonplace and accepted. We suggest that the idea of working within a 'for-profit' business model makes some therapists uncomfortable. It is necessary to acknowledge that placing money and therapy together raises important ethical dilemmas (see Chapters 4 and 5 for further detail). Interactions between financial profit and disadvantage (social/health/mental/physical) or medical needs create challenging and uncomfortable debates. Considering if we can care for our clients, colleagues, commissioners and cash-flow, by necessity has at its centre a strong ethical dimension.

Moving creative arts therapies onto a more financially independent and secure 'for-profit' business model has two distinct but interrelated areas: economics and ethics. We believe that creative arts therapist business owners hold high ethical standards at their core, honed from their time as practising therapists, which can and should be transferred into their business management processes. Therapists who are able to balance the clinical needs of their clients or caseload with the financial sustainability of their business put themselves in a strong position when it comes to long-term development and expansion of therapeutic services.

Tax revenue for funding

The ethical quandary is that all therapy must be funded; without funding we can offer nothing. Governments generally provide funding directly or indirectly, and governments don't always have the revenue to do this as thoroughly as the need might dictate. Governments are reliant on tax revenue to fund services and there are many services demanding funding, with health, education and welfare being the biggest and highest priorities. As governments change and world events evolve, so priorities shift. Funding for therapy is often at the end of a long list of priorities. A healthy revenue base is required to fund many of our jobs. Therapy jobs are often seen as 'extras' and therefore can only be funded if tax revenue first covers basic statutory costs plus public service employment, and if the provision of therapy services is seen as a government priority.

Relying on tax revenue alone means we rely on good economic times. It also means we become dependent on the funding bodies and vulnerable to economic changes. This is fine when the tax income is high, as governments can fund large charities to provide 'free therapy services', and can invest in health and education and create specific initiatives to support marginalised groups. If there is not enough government revenue, funding for therapy and treatment can also be provided by charitable giving. When the economy is doing well, individuals can afford to give to charity. When the economy is under pressure, not only is charitable giving affected, but so too is the way that charitable funds are used. Funding for 'extra' services like creative arts therapies may go toward covering funding cuts to core medical and educational requirements when governments are under pressure (although in hardship periods, support for charitable causes and involvement in food banks, community projects and volunteering also rises, according to the Charities Aid Foundation's (2015) World Giving Index).

In some countries, taxpayers can 'gift' money and receive a tax deduction. The impact of this, called 'Gift Aid' in the UK, may also have unforeseen outcomes for charities who provide therapy services. While Gift Aid may provide funding for therapy services through contract employment, as it is dependent on the amount of money gifted, the government loses tax revenue that could have funded a longer-term position. As an example based on current (2016) United Kingdom law, take a person who pays 40 per cent of their income to tax who wants to give £1000 to a charity they support. The taxpayer indicates they want their donation to benefit from Gift Aid, so the UK government must then provide an additional £250 in Gift Aid, increasing the charitable donation to £1250. If the taxpayer then claims charitable giving tax relief (set at 20%) on their annual tax return, the UK government must forfeit another £250, by way of a reduction in payable tax for the taxpayer.

The net result of this is the UK government has £500 less to spend than it would have had the taxpayer not made their charitable donation. It could be argued that this is not important as the charity now has £1250. However, every penny that is spent in either Gift Aid or tax relief is a penny that governments cannot spend on health, education, defence and all other statutory services and departments. Every £500 the UK government loses as a result of a £1000 donation to charity has either got be made up by other taxpayers or clawed back in cutbacks and cost savings, allowing the government to maintain budgets across all areas.

Creative arts therapists know that consistency, continuity and reliability are at the heart of any successful therapy pathway. These three core clinical principles are likely to dissolve when linked to an operating context which is dependent on grant, gifted or government-related incomes, which rise and fall with the times and can impact access to therapy accordingly. As therapists, we work tirelessly to support our clients' increased autonomy. As a profession, as potential therapy business owners or as self-employed therapists we do all we can to enable clients to be as independent as possible, and move away from a dependency state of mind. Why then are we happy working within a context that fosters a financially dependent culture at the core of what we do? We need to champion our financial independence in much the same way, and value our hard-fought freedom as much as we do with our clients.

Why does this matter? It matters because financial health is part of an ecosystem necessary for creative arts therapies and other psychological therapies to thrive, and for individual therapists as practitioners to survive. Attaining and maintaining individual and organisational financial health is critically important in modern fiscal environments. Offering therapy services that may close or shrink due to a funding cut is potentially unethical and harmful to clients and patients. Creative arts therapists have little control over government budgets; however, we can be proactive in controlling the financial health of our own businesses and lives, especially as reliance on government-funded positions may not be an option in the future.

Raising our own revenue for funding

One positive way that creative arts therapists can support government budgets is by running successful for-profit businesses that pay tax. In addition to this, they can also build local communities through employment and spending in other small businesses. This healthy model should not be underestimated. It stimulates economies, creates jobs and enriches local communities. The Small Business and Entrepreneurship Council in America (2016) stated that small businesses were the incubators for innovation and employment growth during the GFC recovery. They also continue to play a vital role in the economy of the United States, producing 46 per cent of the private non-agricultural GDP in 2008. Small businesses play a significant role in the Australian (Reserve Bank of Australia 2012) and UK economy as well, accounting for almost half of employment in the private non-financial sector and over a third of production.

These small businesses that work in the 'for-profit' space provide revenue for government spending via the tax they pay on the profits they generate. In the UK this is called Corporation Tax. This tax goes to the government who redistribute it as they see fit, and some of this money goes back into the system to fund health and community care, roads, education, defence and other core services. Charities and other tax-exempt business models are exempt from paying tax and are typically reliant on government funding. While the largest national charities do vital work in society, their tax-exempt status means that money essentially only goes to them, often in the form of central government grants, without a 'completing of the circle' in the form of a tax payment back to central government. National charities and other tax-exempt organisations are often managing annual turnovers in excess of £100 million, and are operated in every way like a large multi-million pound organisation should be, except with a hugely advantageous tax position. In this way, it could be argued that these organisations being tax exempt actually reduces the amount of money that governments have to spend on statutory services, even though their charitable work adds immense value to society as a whole.

In light of this, there is a clear need for building better understanding around how business and profit work, to increase business education and financial resilience within our professions and to view this in a larger ecosystem of financial health. We work hard to instil resilience in our clients; creating financial resilience to underpin our work should be equally important.

Valuing therapy in financial terms

In order for therapy to hold a value in the market, it has to be valued in terms of what it offers, but also what it returns. This is sometimes a tricky concept to grasp. Therapists add great value in terms of quality-of-life (QOL) indicators and socio-emotional gains that are often difficult to place in terms of economics via standard cost–benefit analyses. As clinicians we are very good at outlining for people the therapeutic returns of intervention, but what are the cost–benefits of our work? Can we measure the positive financial impact that therapy has on healthcare services? In 2013, The George Center for Music Therapy, an American music therapy centre, compiled results from three cost–benefit analyses of music therapy, and found that in the three settings (hospices, hospitals and neonatal intensive care units) music therapy led to a dramatic reduction in the overall cost of treatments. There was a positive impact on length of stay in hospital as well as a reduction in the need for certain drugs. Their report showed a clear case that in these clinical settings music therapy could have a positive benefit for patients, as well as provide a cost benefit for the health institute as a whole (The George Center for Music Therapy, 2013). In other countries, although this work is in its infancy, social cost–benefit analyses (SCBA) of therapy services are starting to emerge. Looking across other sectors, including health at work, SCBA are more common, and highlight benefits to the participant as well as to governments in terms of reducing healthcare spending (Cancelliere *et al.* 2011; Goetzel & Ozminkowski 2008).

Statistics about worldwide therapy services are few and far between. An internet search of creative arts therapies training courses suggested there were about 180 courses around the world (HotCoursesAbroad 2016). However, detailed statistics on fully qualified professionals are harder to find and accurately verify. In a 2012 survey, The World Federation of Music Therapy (2012) suggested there were approximately 14,623 music therapists practising around the world; 4500 of these were practising in the USA (a number of countries had not submitted figures, so weren't included in the survey). A 2016 Freedom of Information request in the UK, via the Health and Care Professions Council (HCPC 2016), highlighted 3881 creative arts therapists registered to practise in the UK. An Australian survey recently reported that there are 481 registered music therapists in the country. The majority of these work between 10 and 19 hours per week and earn between USD $40,000 and $59,000 per annum (Australian Music Therapy Association 2016). With core data on the therapy profession in such short supply, how can we begin to make a reasonable assessment of its value, and the financial contribution it makes to the global economy?

In 2014 the United Nations International Labour Organization (ILO) tried to calculate the average global wage (ILO 2015), taking into account the differences in currency values, hourly rates and a wealth of other 'balancing data'. The ILO uses a 'purchasing power parity' (PPP) dollar rate, which seeks to provide a useful comparative measurement between different economies' wages. Their findings suggest that the average wage in 2014 was $16,100. If we use the Australian Music Therapy Association (AMTA) and the World Federation of Music Therapy data and assume that all 14,623 music therapists worked on average 2.5 days per week, we get an incredibly rough estimate of the economic contribution of the music therapy profession to global GDP of USD $117.7million. It's the equivalent of music therapists contributing 0.156% to global GDP, which in 2016 was estimated to be USD $74 trillion dollars (World Bank 2016). This is like contributing roughly an eighth of an apple towards a pile of 10,000 apples. It is clear that before we can understand the economic value of our work, which should include cost–benefit analyses of our day-to-day therapy work with patients, the therapy profession needs much better data on a range of core areas. Collaborating with universities and PhD programmes may be a way to get this process started.

The future

No one can predict where the future will take us, but we can learn from the past. Financial funding models have changed over the past decade as governments' revenue bases have declined and while expenditure demands continue to increase. While we can assume some government funding will continue into the future, we should also pursue alternative funding models (Abad & Williams 2009). New funding models and ethical paradigms may need to be forged in order to ensure that therapy professions are sustainable, regardless of the economics of the time. Research- and practice-based ideas of self-sustaining methodologies are becoming increasingly more common. The work of Professor Katrina Skewes McFerran and Dr Daphne Rickson within the music therapy profession have been particularly insightful in providing ways that clinical and service development models can (and should) create self-sustaining contexts. In the same way that these approaches have had to take responsibility for the impact (both positive and negative) of expert-led or withdrawal models of therapy, we may now have to really think about, and be responsible for, the impact that our relationship with money has on us as individuals and on our profession.

Within the therapy professions, could utilising a healthy 'for-profit' model have the potential to align the financial context with the therapeutic content? Both strive for wellness, health, independence and the ability to make choices and respond with self-agency. In this model both context and content are moving in the same direction. It would be interesting to speculate on how this may affect the provision, access and standing of a range of therapeutic approaches in the world. Does the American experience, where the highest number of self-employed and for-profit therapy businesses exist, tell us something and suggest an opportunity? And how does the ethical heart of the therapist relate to the work of developing a successful business?

Conclusion

Placing money and therapy together raises important ethical dilemmas and uncomfortable questions. We believe that the creative arts professions need to start investigating this area with as much clarity and integrity as we use when researching our clinical practice areas. It's time we started to consider whether the economic context of our work might impact the emerging models of practice and client outcomes in their widest sense. We are guided by the general ethical principle of 'do no harm', and we work with the client's best interest as our foremost priority. The area of 'best interests' has expanded over the years to include communities, families, organisations and much more within the emerging ecological models. We believe this should now start to include economic health as well. Many ethical guidelines, such as the European Music Therapy Confederation (2005), refer specifically to economic matters:

> The music therapist shall be aware of the degree of dependency inherent to a therapeutic relationship. (S)he shall in no circumstance act in order to satisfy her/his own personal interests (e.g. emotional, sexual, social, or economic interests).

As we take steps towards a new relationship with the financial context of our work, some of the ethical issues that the profession and individual therapists may need to address, which are discussed further in other chapters in this book, include:

- How can we justify earning a living from people who are unwell and need our help?

- How can we reliably and responsibly advertise and market our services?

- How can we maintain the integrity of time-limited treatment plans when our source of revenue ceases when treatment stops?

- How do we employ ourselves, our colleagues and friends?

Looking more widely across related areas, there are many examples of professions allied to health and medicine that operate within a for-profit context and have a strong ethical orientation that we could learn from, and who already operate successfully in the marketplace. In healthcare services we can include private healthcare/hospitals, physiotherapists, psychologists, wheelchair manufacturers and other areas of support, to name a few.

There seems clear evidence that the for-profit sector requires further attention and exploration in how it can create income and jobs within therapy, provide for our personal needs as well as the needs of our clients, and contribute to the economic growth of our communities.

References

Abad, V. and Williams, K. (2009). Funding and employment conditions: Critical issues for Australian music therapy beyond 2009. *Australian Music Therapy Association*, 20 (special edition), 56–62.

Australian Music Therapy Association (2016). *My Profession My Voice Workforce Census*. Retrieved from www.austmta.org.au/brochure/amta-workforce-census on 17 January 2017.

Bruscia, K.E. (1998). *Defining Music Therapy* (2nd edition). Gilsum, NH: Barcelona Publishers.

Cancelliere, C., Cassidy, J.D., Ammendolia, C. and Côté, P. (2011). Are workplace health promotion programs effective at improving presenteeism in workers? A systematic review and best evidence synthesis of the literature. *BMC Public Health*, 11, 395.

Chlan, L. (1998). Effectiveness of a music therapy intervention on relaxation and anxiety for patients receiving ventilatory assistance. *Heart Lung*, 27, 3, 169–176.

Charities Aid Foundation (2015). *CAF World Giving Index 2015: A Global View of Giving Trends*. Retrieved from https://www.cafonline.org/docs/default-source/about-us-publications/caf_worldgivingindex2015_report.pdf?sfvrsn=2 on 10 January 2017.

Davies, C., Knuiman, M. and Rosenberg, M. (2016). The art of being mentally healthy: A study to quantify the relationship between recreational arts engagement and mental well-being in the general population. *BMC Public Health, BMC Series – Open, Inclusive and Trusted*, 16, 15. doi: 10.1186/s12889-015-2672-7.

Davies, C., Rosenberg, M., Knuiman, M., Ferguson, R., Pikora, T. and Slatter, N. (2012). Defining arts engagement for population-based health research: Art forms, activities and level of engagement. *Arts Health*, 4, 3, 203–216.

Edwards, J. (2011). A music and health perspective on music's perceived 'goodness'. *Nordic Journal of Music Therapy*, 20, 1, 90–101.

European Music Therapy Confederation (2005). *Ethical Code*. Retrieved from http://emtc-eu.com/ethical-code on 24 November 2016.

George Center for Music Therapy (2013). *Three Studies on the Cost Benefit of Music Therapy*. Retrieved from http://www.thegeorgecenter.com/2013/06/05/3-studies-on-the-cost-benefits-of-music-therapy on 13 March 2017.

Goetzel, R.Z. and Ozminkowski, R.J. (2008). The health and cost benefits of work site health-promotion programs. *Annual Rev Public Health*, 29, 303–323.

Guzzetta, C.E. (1989) Effects of relaxation and music therapy on patients in a coronary care unit with presumptive acute myocardial infarction. *Heart and Lung*, 18, 6, 609–616.

HCPC (2016). Retrieved from www.hcpc-uk.co.uk/assets/documents/10004FBFMusic DramaandArtsTherapists2000-2015.pdf on 24 November 2016.

HotCoursesAbroad (2016). Retrieved from www.hotcoursesabroad.com.

International Labour Organization (2015). *Global Wage Report 2014/15*. Retrieved from www.ilo.org/wcmsp5/groups/public/---dgreports/---dcomm/---publ/documents/publication/wcms_324839.pdf on 24 November 2016.

Korkki (2012) Food banks expand beyond hunger. *New York Times* (8 November). Retrieved from www.nytimes.com/2012/11/09/giving/food-banks-mission-expands-to-nutrition-and-education.html?_r=0 on 24 November 2016.

Krout, R.E. (2006). Music listening to facilitate relaxation and promote wellness: Integrated aspects of our neurophysiological responses to music. *Arts Psychotherapy*, 34, 2, 134–141.

McNicoll, A. (2015). *Mental health trust funding down 8% from 2010 despite coalition's drive for parity of esteem*. Community Care, 20 March. Retrieved from www.communitycare.co.uk/2015/03/20/mental-health-trust-funding-8-since-2010-despite-coalitions-drive-parity-esteem on 24 November 2016.

NCVO (2013). *Counting the Cuts: The Impact of Spending Cuts on the UK Voluntary and Community Sector*. Retrieved from www.ncvo.org.uk/images/documents/policy_and_research/localism/counting_the_cuts.pdf on 10 January 2017.

Reserve Bank of Australia (2012). *Small Business: An Economic Overview*. Retrieved from www.rba.gov.au/publications/workshops/other/small-bus-fin-roundtable-2012/pdf/01-overview.pdf on 24 November 2016.

Romo, R. and Gifford, L. (2007). A cost-benefit analysis of music therapy in a home hospice. *Nursing Economics*, 25, 6, 353–358.

Sandel, S.L., Judge, J.O., Landry, N., Faria, L., Ouellette, R. and Majczak, M. (2005). Dance and movement program improves quality-of-life measures in breast cancer survivors. *Cancer Nurse*, 28, 4, 301–309.

Small Business and Entrepreneurship Council (2016). *Small Business Facts & Data*. Retrieved from http://sbecouncil.org/about-us/facts-and-data on 24 November 2016.

Staricoff, R.L. (2006). Arts in health: The value of evaluation. *Journal of the Royal Society for the Promotion of Health*, 126, 3, 116–120.

Stuckey, H. L. and Nobel, J. (2010). The connection between art, healing, and public health: A review of current literature. *American Journal of Public Health*, 100, 2, 254–263.

Tadeo, M. and Duarte, E. (2016). *Spain runs out of workers with almost 5 million unemployed*. Bloomberg, 1 July. Retrieved from www.bloomberg.com/news/articles/2016-07-01/spain-is-running-out-of-workers-with-almost-5-million-unemployed on 24 November 2016.

Winnicott, D.W. (1973). *The Child, the Family, and the Outside World*. Middlesex: Penguin Psychology.

World Bank (2016). *Gross Domestic Product 2015.* Retrieved from http://databank. worldbank.org/data/download/GDP.pdf on 10 January 2017.

World Federation of Music Therapy (2012). *Accreditation & Certification Commission: Music Therapy Certifications and Licenses Worldwide.* Retrieved from www.wfmt. info/WFMT/Accreditation_and_Certification_1_files/Music%20Therapy%20 Certifications%202012.pdf on 10 January 2017.

CHAPTER 2

Entrepreneuring in Arts Therapies
Not Just Making a Swift Buck
Alison Ledger

Introduction

This chapter stems from my PhD research in music therapy (Ledger 2010), in which I explored music therapists' experiences of developing new services. In this research, I collected rich narratives of service development from 11 music therapists from five countries and undertook fieldwork to observe a music therapist in the start-up phase. These music therapists conveyed strong feelings of isolation, insecurity and uncertainty in developing services, and reported challenges such as role ambiguity and resistance from other workers. Literature about management and organisational change was particularly valuable for understanding these experiences and I have continued to apply management theory in reflecting on music therapy work (Ledger, Edwards, & Morley 2013).

One interesting finding from my PhD study was that music therapists distanced themselves from the business world and expressed uncertainty about what they needed to do to achieve financial security. At the same time, the music therapists in my study displayed qualities commonly attributed to entrepreneurs, such as creativity, passion and persistence (Kuratko 2014; Lumsdaine & Binks 2009). This has led me to wonder why arts therapists may be reluctant to adopt an entrepreneurial identity and I have started to consider the fit between understandings of entrepreneurship and arts therapy practice.

This chapter provides a brief history of the field of entrepreneurship, including the shift in interest from the individual entrepreneur to the entrepreneuring process. I then provide examples from my PhD research to show how arts therapists may be engaged in entrepreneuring processes, whether developing a business or working in a more established post. Rather than suggesting arts therapists learn about entrepreneurship, I propose that a focus on *entrepreneuring* may sit comfortably with arts therapists and encourage arts therapists to attend to their particular business contexts.

Background

Entrepreneurship is a diverse field occupied by a range of disciplines, terminology, definitions, research methods, schools of thought, and interests (Bridge & O'Neill 2013; Down 2010; Kuratko 2014). Early understandings of entrepreneurship were limited to the process of starting or running a small business; however, broader understandings of entrepreneurship have since emerged (Bridge & O'Neill 2013). Entrepreneurship now often refers to any 'creative contribution in the world of work' (Northern Ireland Government 2003, p.5) and a way of dealing with the uncertainty and complexity of modern-day life (Bridge & O'Neill 2013). The expansion of entrepreneurship to different countries and contexts has been described as an 'entrepreneurial revolution' (Kuratko 2014, p.4) and entrepreneurship is frequently promoted as a desirable ethos, mind-set, or way of life (Bridge & O'Neill 2013; Down 2010; Kuratko 2014). Most current definitions of entrepreneurship emphasise newness, change, risk management and a tolerance of ambiguity. For example, Kuratko (2014) defines entrepreneurship as:

> a dynamic process of vision, change, and creation. It requires an application of energy and passion toward the creation and implementation of new ideas and creative solutions. Essential ingredients include the willingness to take calculated risks – in terms of time, equity, or career; the ability to formulate an effective venture team; the creative skill to marshal needed resources; the fundamental skill of building a solid business plan; and finally, the vision to recognize opportunity where others see chaos, contradiction, and confusion. (p.5)

Much research about entrepreneurship has aimed to identify the particular behaviours, attributes, skills, values and beliefs of entrepreneurs and to predict entrepreneurial success (Bridge & O'Neill 2013; Down 2010). This research has led to the identification of common entrepreneurial traits, such as creativity, autonomy, perseverance and determination (Bridge & O'Neill 2013; Down 2010; Kuratko 2014). Arts therapists, who often work as sole and pioneering practitioners and for whom creativity is fundamental, may view these traits as desirable. However, entrepreneurship is often associated with traits that arts therapists may not view as positively, such as aggressiveness, competitiveness and a desire for achievement in terms of economic growth (Down 2010; Kuratko 2014). These traits may be less acceptable for workers trained to build client-centred relationships, develop supportive aims and focus on achieving therapeutic outcomes. Perhaps it is for this reason that the music therapists in my study seemed reluctant to identify as an entrepreneur.

A more recent approach to studying entrepreneurship is the creative process or social construction approach (Down 2010). While the dominant trait-based approach to studying entrepreneurship focuses on the individual entrepreneur, the creative process approach places greater emphasis on the context in which entrepreneurship behaviour takes place. Scholars such as Down (2010) and Steyaert (2007) recognise that understandings of entrepreneurship are constantly changing and that the extent to which someone is described or describes themselves as an entrepreneur depends on the time and place. Rather than seeing entrepreneurship as a fixed trait possessed by individuals, these scholars understand entrepreneurship as a 'more fluid and emergent process combining different behaviours, thinking and identity constructions in a social process' (Down 2010, p.68). According to this processual understanding, a range of situations may be conducive or obstructive to entrepreneuring, including cultural, economic, personal or historical circumstances (Down 2010).

The creative process approach to entrepreneurship resonates with my analysis of music therapists' experiences, which highlighted the importance of context in music therapy service development (Ledger 2010). Music therapists' experiences depended on aspects such as an organisation's history, culture and financial systems. Furthermore, I suspect that a focus on entrepreneuring may be more acceptable to arts therapists who are less inclined to convey an entrepreneurial identity. I wonder whether an entrepreneurial identity may be less legitimate for therapists who have a strong helper identity and for whom therapeutic relationships are critical. For this reason, in this chapter I have decided to focus on ways in which arts therapists may be engaged in processes of entrepreneuring, irrespective of whether the arts therapist is employed or self-employed. I give particular attention to the ways in which entrepreneuring in arts therapies may be helped or hindered by the particular context, to promote further awareness of this critical feature of arts therapy business development. The reader's context may be a place of employment or their own business; in either case, the focus is on expanding services.

Entrepreneuring in music therapy

While the music therapists in my study did not identify as entrepreneurs, their stories and actions indicated that they were involved in processes of entrepreneuring. Four common processes are described here: identifying opportunities and barriers, building relationships, being creative and flexible, and maintaining passion and persistence. Case examples are provided to further illustrate these processes and to highlight the impact of context on arts therapy business development. Therapists' names have been changed and countries have been omitted to preserve anonymity.

Identifying opportunities and barriers

Music therapy developers in my study were commonly concerned with identifying opportunities and barriers to service growth. Their stories explained how they identified niches for introducing new services and were careful to push for development at the right time. Some described how they had identified ways that music therapy could meet a gap or enhance existing services, while others recounted how they had identified an opportunity to push for more resources. Bonnie, for example, recalled how she identified an opportunity to ask for a second music therapy position in mental health.

> After a couple of years of successful music therapy implementation, Bonnie was beginning to feel confident in her abilities and had started to take on music therapy students. She had received positive feedback from staff and patients and had built a strong working relationship with her manager. At this time, Bonnie noted that the hospital was employing other allied health professions staff and she realised this was a prime time to

> ask for a second music therapy position. At the time her manager was enthusiastic about the music therapy service and wanted programmes to continue when the music therapy students left. Bonnie suggested a second music therapy post to her manager, who then raised the idea with the director of nursing, and before too long, a new music therapist was appointed.

Music therapists not only described how they had identified opportunities, but also how they had recognised barriers to further growth. This was particularly evident in Catie's story, in which she described how her position was limited in the current environment.

> Catie hoped to expand music therapy provision to other areas of the children's hospital, but explained that it was not the right time to be putting these plans into action. She doubted the team's acceptance of music therapy and felt that she needed to wait for staff to become more comfortable and familiar with music therapy's contribution. She also recognised that there had been many recent changes in staff and that staff were not ready for additional change. Catie accepted that music therapy growth would be slow and that she would need to wait for changes in the workplace culture.

Both Bonnie and Catie could be seen to be involved in entrepreneuring, albeit at different points in their service development process. Though they had been employed for similar lengths of time, opportunities for growth had appeared in Bonnie's workplace while Catie was waiting for such opportunities to arise.

Building relationships

Building relationships was one of the main themes I identified in my doctoral work, as nearly all of the service development narratives emphasised a need for music therapists to build relationships with other staff. Participants stressed that it was most important to build relationships with people who had the power to influence their economic survival. Most often, this was a staff member in a position of power, such as a hospital or service manager or a trusted and respected member of staff. Brad in particular emphasised the importance of building mutually beneficial relationships with managers and marketers.

After many years working in palliative care, Brad had learned the importance of give and take in building relationships with managers and marketers. He found ways to not only secure the resources needed for a high-quality music therapy service, but also meet the business needs of the hospice where he worked. He gave music therapy presentations to the public and healthcare community, which helped to establish a unique selling point for the hospice. Hospice marketers attributed business growth to the additional music therapy service. In addition, Brad recognised that the hospice was subject to funding cuts and exercised care when making requests for further resources. His advice was to settle on one wish a year and make it a good one.

While Brad reflected on the importance of building relationships with managers and marketers, Marion perceived that she needed to build relationships with other members of the multidisciplinary healthcare team.

When Marion started work for a mental health service, she encountered new ways of working, experienced little team support, and faced an uncertain future. She spent two weeks meeting various members of staff to understand others' priorities and the different ways people worked. Each unit had a different consultant, with a distinct style of practice and approach to organising the multidisciplinary team. It was therefore important to spend time getting to know different team members, to understand how music therapy could best fit in. Through drinking many cups of tea and listening to staff, she developed a music therapy service which was accessible and responsive to both staff and service users' needs.

While Brad and Marion described how they had built relationships with staff, music therapists also built relationships with people who were not in traditional positions of power. For example, those working in children's services described how parents had played an important role in advocating and securing funding for a music therapist and developing a music therapy service that met clients' needs. The locations of power are likely to depend on the particular work context and a key entrepreneuring process may be identifying whose buy-in is essential.

Being creative and flexible

Being creative and flexible was another entrepreneuring process that music therapists were involved in. Music therapists found themselves working in ways they had not expected and deviating from the methods and approaches they were most familiar with from their training. Through being flexible, they created services to meet the needs, demands and expectations of managers, staff and clients. This was most notable in Rachel's story, when she described how her practice had deviated from her training.

Rachel was trained in psychodynamic approaches to music therapy and mostly used improvisational methods in her previous work. When she started work with children on a rehabilitation ward, children, parents and staff expected her to use pre-composed music, such as well-known children's songs and music currently in the charts. She began to experiment with recreative methods, including the use of recorded music. These different forms of music were highly effective in engaging the children, promoting social interaction, supporting treatment goals, and involving parents and staff in music therapy implementation. Rachel questioned whether she was still practising music therapy while exploring these new therapy approaches. However, she concluded that she remained faithful to her training when she monitored therapeutic outcomes and continued to reflect on the psychodynamic aspects of her work.

Rachel's story shows how music therapists may need to decide which aspects of their practice are essential and which aspects they are willing to compromise on. Different client groups (for example, managers, adult service users, children or parents) are likely to have different hopes and expectations of music therapy than trained music therapists. Music therapists may therefore need to be flexible when entering negotiations and seeking and securing employment.

Maintaining passion and persistence

Almost all of the music therapists in my study experienced frustrations and setbacks. Music therapists recalled waxes and wanes in financial and managerial support, the number of music therapy hours and posts, and levels of staff resistance to music therapy. However, music therapists worked hard to maintain and convey their initial enthusiasm and gained a sense of achievement by overcoming challenges. One such music therapist was Margot, who persisted in the face of low staff morale, management complications and a lack of team support.

> When Margot started in the mental health unit, other staff placed little value on music therapy and even told her, 'We don't need you.' Little by little, she built up small pockets of support, through giving music therapy presentations and involving staff in music therapy work. A couple of years later, Margot prepared a business proposal for a permanent music therapy post, which was approved by the executive group. However, severe financial constraints meant that the post was later placed on a wish list. Although this situation could be viewed as a setback, Margot held hope that a permanent post would eventually be created and gained immediate rewards from seeing patients and music therapy students benefit from the service she was currently providing. Margot could still see opportunities for growth and intended to continue fighting for them.

While Margot was remaining optimistic, other music therapists struggled to maintain passion and persistence. One final process that could be understood as entrepreneuring is the process of deciding to withdraw a music therapy service and start up somewhere new. At the time of my study, Michelle was coming to the conclusion that she was unable to persist and it was time to leave to seek opportunities elsewhere.

> Michelle had worked tirelessly as a music therapist in a children's hospital for over ten years. In that time, she had seen other music therapy staff come and go, expansion and reduction in music therapy services, increases and decreases in funding. After years of writing grant applications, endless submissions and little internal funding, Michelle was beginning to run out of steam. The rewards of working with children and their families were no longer enough to sustain her enthusiasm. She was beginning to concede that it was time to say goodbye and to start up a new business venture.

Although this may seem like a negative note to finish on, recognising the time to move on may be an important entrepreneuring process that music therapists experience. Joanne Loewy (2001) has encouraged music therapists to build work only where there is support for growth, and it should be noted that Michelle has continued to develop a successful music therapy business since leaving the hospital.

Conclusion

Arts therapists may not think of themselves as entrepreneurs. I know that I never thought of myself as an entrepreneur, even when self-employed, sub-contracting or working on part-time or temporary music therapy contracts. I understood increases of hours or pay as signs that my contribution to care was valued, not as an indication of economic success. I never entered the music therapy profession to make money; I only wanted to help people and spend my working life doing something I enjoyed and found rewarding. I suspect many arts therapists think about their work in similar ways.

However, arts therapists may be involved in processes of entrepreneuring by contributing to service development and business growth. This chapter highlighted four ways in which arts therapists may be involved in entrepreneuring: identifying opportunities and barriers, building relationships, being creative and flexible, and maintaining passion and persistence. These are just a few examples, as entrepreneuring processes are likely to depend on the context, including whether the arts therapist is self-employed or working as an employee, the way a service is organised and funded, the workplace culture, and the specific client group. Additionally, arts therapists may develop new ways of entrepreneuring in response to the particular barriers and affordances present in their work or business context.

I propose that the creative process approach to entrepreneuring offers ways of understanding arts therapy practice and how arts therapy businesses and services grow. The reduced emphasis on the individual entrepreneur may suit arts therapists who do not identify with entrepreneurial traits. Furthermore, the creative process approach highlights the key role of context in business growth. As emphasised in this chapter, an awareness of context is critical for developing valuable arts therapy work that meets clients' needs.

Go and do it!
Exercise 1: Map out the terrain

This chapter emphasised the importance of considering your particular business context. This first exercise requires you to think about opportunities and barriers to arts therapy business development. First, spend some time identifying who has the power to influence your economic survival and who has an interest in seeing your business grow. It may be helpful to place these people on a stakeholder analysis grid, as in Figure 2.1:

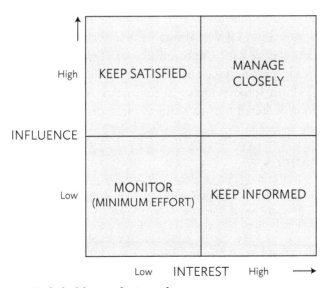

Figure 2.1 Stakeholder analysis grid
(Imperial College London 2016)

This work will help you to ascertain who it is most important to build relationships with. You should spend more time and energy building relationships with those placed in the high-influence half and worry less about building relationships with those who are least influential and unlikely to invest in the growth of your business.

Second, think about the various situational factors that are likely to affect your business survival and growth (for example, cultural, economic, personal or historical factors). You may find it helpful to make two lists – opportunities and barriers. What resources are available for taking advantage of opportunities and overcoming barriers? How can you maintain passion and persistence when faced with challenges or disappointments?

Exercise 2: Meeting clients' needs

Being creative and flexible was one example of an entrepreneuring process. You will need to meet clients' needs in order to obtain and maintain business. Clients may be expecting a different service to what you plan to deliver (based on your arts therapy training and experience).

This exercise aims to prepare you for flexibility in arts therapy service provision. Spend a few weeks thinking about what is essential to the client and which aspects of your arts therapy practice meet those needs. After reflecting on this for some time, write down what it is that your business will always offer and the possible directions the therapy service can take to meet your clients' needs. This work will not only prepare you for upcoming business negotiations, but also be helpful for developing a distinctive service and designing promotional material such as business cards and information leaflets.

References

Bridge, S. and O'Neill, K. (2013). *Understanding Enterprise Entrepreneurship and Small Business* (4th edition). Basingstoke: Palgrave Macmillan.

Down, S. (2010). *Enterprise, Entrepreneurship and Small Business.* London: Sage.

Imperial College London. (2016). *Project Stakeholder Analysis.* Retrieved from https://workspace.imperial.ac.uk/projectmanagement/public/Templates%20for%20download/Stakeholder%20analysis.doc on 11 August 2015.

Kuratko, D.F. (2014). *Introduction to Entrepreneurship* (9th edition). Australia: Cengage Learning.

Ledger, A. (2010). *Am I a founder or am I a fraud? Music therapists' experiences of developing services in healthcare organizations.* Unpublished doctoral thesis, University of Limerick, Limerick.

Ledger, A., Edwards, J. and Morley, M. (2013). A change management perspective on the introduction of music therapy to interprofessional teams. *Journal of Health Organization and Management,* 27, 6, 714–732.

Loewy, J.V. (2001). Building bridges in team centred care. *Australian Journal of Music Therapy,* 12, 3–12.

Lumsdaine, E. and Binks, M. (2009). *Entrepreneurship from Creativity to Innovation: Thinking Skills for a Changing World.* Victoria, BC: Trafford.

Northern Ireland Government (2003). *Entrepreneurship and Education Action Plan.* Belfast: Departments of Enterprise, Trade and Investment (DETI), Education (DE) and Employment and Learning (DEL).

Steyaert, C. (2007). 'Entrepreneuring' as a conceptual attractor? A review of process theories in 20 years of entrepreneurship studies. *Entrepreneurship and Regional Development,* 19, 6, 453–477.

CHAPTER 3

RAILE – Building a Win-Win Business Model for Therapy

Vicky Abad and Daniel Thomas

Introduction

Every day, across the world, when a client starts a therapy session, the therapist begins listening to and processing a range of information. This includes non-verbal cues such as body language, facial expressions, the slogan on a t-shirt they wear, which chair or part of the room they go to, the client's breathing rate, as well as any verbal or musical/artistic/dramatic cues. The therapist may say hello, start to play music or improvise a way to make an initial connection. As the client acknowledges the therapist, either with words or through sound or gesture, the therapist is attuning to their mood or feeling state. If the client ignores the therapist but starts to interact with an instrument, or play with clay, or simply looks out of a window, the therapist is attuned to them and ever present and fully focused in the here-and-now – they remain resilient and available no matter what. The therapist may improvise by listening, reflecting, interacting musically, attuning to meet the client in the moment. The client may begin using a creative modality with confidence and delight. Or they may sit nervously and fidget. The therapist may start to wonder about how the client is feeling, they start to empathise with them... wondering, listening, adapting.

Our everyday practice as therapists is borne from years of initial study and training, and once qualified we hone these core clinical skills in the real world with real people. We become so adept at using these skills that their once clunky application becomes a (mostly) seamless and quiet inner process that turns on and off without much conscious awareness.

These core clinical skills that therapists are already good at are powerful and transferrable skills that can be equally useful in the business space. We hope this chapter will plant some seeds for you to go away and reflect and act upon.

While starting a business requires a different set of skills (see Chapters 2 and 6 for more details), transferrable core therapy skills can be applied to build a thriving business. In this chapter, we examine which skills are transferrable, and introduce a new concept that highlights how you can apply these skills in your therapy business today.

Transferrable skills

Transferrable skills are those you develop in one situation or setting that can be transferred to another. You develop these throughout your life, as part of your education, community roles and family roles. In the modern employment world employers are looking for key transferrable skills that employees bring with them. For you, this means being able to demonstrate to commissioners and those making funding decisions that you have skills that can be transferred to this new setting. These can be both personal and professional.

The Queensland University of Technology have outlined the following as personal transferrable skills (PTS):

- communication skills

- teamwork skills

- managing and organising skills

- problem-solving skills.

(QUT 2016)

We believe that in addition to these PTS, you have a set of core clinical skills that strengthen your PTS and can help you to build successful businesses. These skills are: resilience, attunement, improvisation, listening and empathy (RAILE). While we understand their value within a clinical/therapeutic setting, RAILE skills are also at the core of building successful 'win-win' relationships within the realm of business or service development.

First, let's look at how these strengthen your PTS and therefore make you a stronger employment and business candidate:

- *Communication skills:* Good communicators are those who listen well, and hear what is actually being said so that they may 'listen between the lines'. Good communicators listen and watch for verbal and non-verbal cues.

- *Teamwork skills*: Teamwork requires great listening skills, being in tune with your team members, having the ability to work flexibly with the team, and the capacity to show empathy to other people's ideas or initiatives.

- *Managing and organising skills*: Managing and organising skills require you to be resilient. It is not easy to manage people, accounts, organisations, and their expectations, budgets, hopes and fears. You first and foremost need a resilient person who is attuned to the needs of the organisation and its people – its employees and its clients. These needs are often very different, and to meet all of these differing needs you need someone creative and flexible in their management approach.

- *Problem-solving skills:* Problem-solving skills require a similar resilient approach. When it comes to therapy and funding there are many problems to solve. A resilient person is required to navigate these waters and lead a team of people. This person needs to be in tune with both the stakeholders and the clients, show empathy to their differing needs and be able to hear what they are all saying, often at the same time. A creative approach is required to manage their wants and needs and solve the problems in positive ways. Creative arts therapists have all of these skills, honed not only through their life experiences but through their very specific and thorough training.

Can therapists use these core clinical skills within a business framework to improve relationships with purchasers of therapy services (commissioners), and improve outcomes for clients and themselves at the same time? We believe so. We also believe they are necessary to build equitable, ethical and empirical business models, for the provision of therapeutic services generally and the creative arts therapies specifically. Table 3.1 shows how RAILE skills are applicable to PTS skills. We have emphasised the more applicable skills, although there is an overlap across all RAILE and PTS skills:

Table 3.1 RAILE vs. PTS transferrable skills

Personal transferrable skill	RAILE transferrable skill
Communication skills	Attunement Listening
Teamwork skills	Attunement Improvisation Listening Empathy
Managing and organising skills	Resilience Attunement Improvisation Listening Empathy
Problem-solving skills	Resilience Attunement Improvisation Listening Empathy

RAILE – the concept

The conceptualisation of RAILE (Abad & Thomas 2013) developed out of many years as business owners in Australia and the UK, and a chance moment of hearing Daniel Pink, author of *To Sell is Human* (2014), talk on the radio. Hearing Pink discuss sales techniques within an updated 'ABC' framework of Attunement, Buoyancy and Clarity, sounded familiar. Rather than 'Always Be Closing', Pink's recasting of the sales mantra as an adaptive, responsive and playful way of engaging with potential commissioners had much appeal, and appeared to have crossover points to the world of therapy practice. If attunement is attunement, buoyancy is understood to be resilience, clarity is seen as improvisation.

Years of reflecting on what it was we did that worked in therapy and business, and how these complemented each other, started to line up. We began to devise a model that supported therapists to transfer their core clinical skills to a business setting. At its heart is our belief that great therapy and great business are all about creating great relationships. The relationship is the common ground between therapy and business, and between therapist and salesperson. RAILE is the coming together of the following core clinical skills within the context of business/sales and how these core skills interrelate with each other. To recap, they are:

- resilience

- attunement

- improvisation

- listening

- empathy.

RAILE – for sale

As discussed in Chapter 1, many creative arts therapists are uncomfortable with private practice work, where fees are set and money changes hands. Perhaps this is because, ultimately, what you are doing is 'closing the sale', exchanging your service in return for money. Therapists may associate the idea of selling with the outdated pressure sales model of 'sell, sell, sell' (Pink 2014). But the reality is, 'to sell is human' (Pink 2014) and we do it all the time. As therapists, we are always selling our services and our profession. To sell is basically to persuade someone of the merits of what we do, to convince them to join us in a dialogue as we move them with the power of music or drama or art. This happens in the therapy room, on the train, at the dinner party.

Psychologists and social science researchers have now begun to realise that to run a successful business, new qualities are required to replace the stereotyped image of pressure sales. Indeed, in the age of the Google search, buyers of services and products can obtain as much information on an item as the seller has. There is a developing equality in the transaction, and one that we would recognise and positively work towards in the clinical space in terms of informed consent, and collaboration and inclusion in the process of buying/ participating in therapy.

If our core therapeutic skills of resilience, attunement, improvisation and listening are transferred and applied within the sphere of the larger business world with great empathy for the needs of both the client and the commissioner, their importance and value when developing successful creative arts businesses and partnerships can be better seen and understood. Clients, therapists and partner organisations alike benefit from clear financial contexts and boundaries as they allow ethical and appropriate therapy work to take place and put all aspects of our work on sustainable and equitable financial foundations.

RAILE – the model

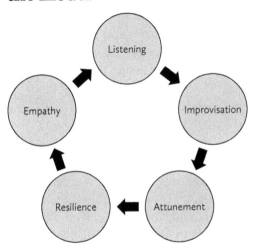

Figure 3.1 RAILE – the model

RAILE starts with resilience, as you must be willing to endure the possibility of rejection. However, in a practical sense, RAILE is underpinned by listening. It takes just one tenth of a second to make a first impression (Willis & Todorov 2006). Even before the therapist has said hello to the commissioner (head teacher, hospital manager, care home coordinator), they have picked up non-verbal signals. As they touch hands to shake they are picking up further physical and sensory cues, with interpretations being made of each other due to the firmness or otherwise of the grip and grasp (Chaplin *et al.* 2000; Donnelly 2015). Listening happens immediately and constantly. Let's explore each element of RAILE in more detail.

Resilience

Resilience is traditionally and commonly viewed as the 'process of adapting well in the face of adversity, trauma, tragedy, threats, or even significant sources of stress – such as family and relationship problems, serious health problems, or workplace and financial stressors. It means "bouncing back" from difficult experiences' (American Psychological Association 2016).

It can be viewed as an umbrella term that describes a number of behaviours, thoughts and actions that can be learned and developed. Another understanding of resilience sees it in light of the person's ability to successfully navigate life events (Masten 2001, 2011) and, as such, choose how they will respond to events as they experience them (Ruksenas 2013). People develop a range of protective factors and risk factors, and those with more protective factors have higher levels of resilience.

Music therapists work with clients to build resilience all of the time (see Docherty *et al.* 2013; Pasiali 2010; Robb *et al.* 2014 for further information). We tap into music's ability to build independence (Abad 2003), nurture self-efficacy (Nicholsen *et al.* 2008), and at the same time build self-regulatory abilities (Winsler, Ducenne & Koury 2011) and support attachment relationships (Abad & Edwards 2004; Abad & Williams 2006, 2007; Edwards 2011; Oldfield 2011).

We believe that music therapists and their creative arts colleagues are excellent at facilitating resilience in their clients, and in themselves. You have made it through many years of dedicated practice and intense training, had to reflect, with great scrutiny, your motivations for becoming a therapist, and had to draw on your personal resources to work in a field that is under-recognised, misunderstood and underfunded. How many times have you had to explain what it is you do? How many grant applications have you written? New position descriptions? How many times have these been knocked back? The list goes on and on. Creative arts therapists draw on resilience in their practice every day to manage themselves, and also to strengthen and empower their clients. We suggest that you can also use this to build your business.

Resilience is required to navigate the many knock-backs, closed doors and hurdles you will have to overcome. But as a creative arts therapist haven't you already had to do this? Resilience in the business world requires the same therapeutic skill of remaining buoyant and strong in the face of adversity.

Attunement

The next core clinical skill we begin using in the RAILE model is attunement. Therapists are very good at tuning in to the needs of their clients. We are tuning in to what makes people tick, what will make them better in the therapy room, what will help sustain them outside of it all of the time. As we mentioned earlier, to sell is to move people, to inspire them to join in a dialogue with you. We are a passionate bunch, and we do this all of the time. We move people with our stories daily; we convince them to join us in a dialogue as we move them with the power of music, art, drama or any other communicative modality.

In the business sense, Pink (2014) describes attunement as 'understanding another person's perspective, getting inside his head, and seeing the world through his eyes…this is done by assuming you are not the one with power' (Pink 2014, p.155). From a therapeutic perspective, Stern refers to attunement behaviours as those which 'recast the event and shift the focus of attention to what is behind the behaviour, to the quality of feeling that is being shared' (Stern 2000, p.142). Both of these descriptions describe the therapy world. As therapists, we never assume a position of power, rather we see ourselves as facilitators, collaborators, and partners in change. The more empowered our clients are, the better the outcomes. We also help our clients become more attuned to themselves, others or events, and facilitate and guide this process as the therapist.

For example, in music therapy, music is often used as a catalyst to help parents attune to their infants (Abad 2011; Creighton, Atherton & Kitamura 2013; Edwards & Abad 2016). When an infant and mother are attuned to each other we see this through musical and dance-like interactions, where they sing and move to, and in time with, each other (Malloch & Trevarthen 2009). Winnicott (1987 [1952]) believed that this ability to tune in with the baby was the key factor that provided the 'good enough' conditions in which a baby develops and thrives. Music therapists use music to support and develop this ability to tune in, in their therapeutic work.

Both Stern (2000) and Pink (2014) are talking about the same process, although in very different contexts. This core therapeutic skill is equally transferrable from relationship-building in therapy to relationship-building in business by being attuned to what the consumer wants, whether this be the privately paying client or the commissioner funding the therapy position. In business, the more attuned we are, the more we understand what is motivating the client (the commissioner) and what their needs are, the better we will be at meeting this need. We have to be attuned to what the need is in order to provide a solution. And we have to be ready to be flexible in order to meet it.

Improvisation

In the business world, having the ability to improvise without preparation and make something from whatever is available is a valuable skill to have. This skill means you can be flexible in meeting the needs of your client, the commissioner, who you are now attuned to and whose needs you now know, but you may or may not have the resources required. Instead of going in with an inflexible plan, if you have the ability to adapt, to respond, to create, you are more likely to meet that need.

In the clinical space we mostly think of improvisation in musical terms. Tony Wigram defined clinical musical improvisation as 'the use of musical improvisation in an environment of trust and support established to meet the needs of clients' (Wigram 2004, p.37). However, we would argue that creative arts therapists are excellent improvisers in many aspects of their jobs. How often have you turned up to a school to find they don't have the appropriate amount of equipment to run your group, and you make do anyway? Or you turn up at a nursing home job to be told there are 200 residents and they would like you to provide music therapy for all the clients in your six-hour shift? Are you going to turn around and leave? No! You are going to improvise and make do with what you have. Of course we wouldn't advocate providing music therapy services to 200 residents in one day, but saying 'No' is going to shut that door immediately. The ability to improvise is going to mean you get in the door, you are flexible with the services you can realistically provide and creative with your responses to management on how better you could service their needs with more hours or fewer clients. Saying 'No, but' to a difficult and unforeseen turn in events shuts down conversation. Saying 'Yes, and' starts conversations, it opens doors and opportunities, and improvising allows you to explore them. Through active listening while improvising, we can then start to piece together a solution. The Latin word 'improvisus' means 'unforeseen', and improvisation happens when you can't see the end goal but you keep moving ahead, dealing with obstacles in a creative way (Vocabulary.com n.d.).

Listening

To be a good seller you need to be a better listener. This skill is at the very heart of RAILE. You need to hear what people want, hear the information often hidden in the detail. An informed listener incorporates space and reflection and while doing so finds ways to address the listener's concerns. Therapists are excellent listeners. We have highly developed listening and reflecting skills. Active listening leads to innovative outcomes.

In a business sense, how can we find the funds to create the space to allow the therapy to happen? When a commissioner (teacher, social worker, etc.) says they can't afford an arts therapist right now, do you hear 'we can't afford a therapist' or do you hear 'right now'? An active listener hears, reflects, responds, and often in a creative way. This creative response is rooted in the therapist's capacity for resilience – not being afraid of rejection – and is then informed by their willingness to continue to be available in the conversation. By acknowledging 'what is so/the current situation' and looking for a solution or a 'next step', both the therapist and the commissioner feel understood and validated.

Expanding on the example above, if we can hear 'right now', the therapist could then ask the commissioner, 'Right now suggests that in the future the current pressure on budgets may change – are you one of the main budget holders in the organisation?' Keeping the conversation alive, while acknowledging the presented difficulty, also allows the therapist to identify who controls the therapy budget and who to talk to in the future. This is the process of building relationships through our active therapeutic listening skills. By focusing on what is important, that is, developing the relationship with the person you're talking to, rather than on the outcome you want (a job/a therapy contract), you, the therapist, are more likely to secure a long-term relationship with the commissioner and give them the experience of being heard/listened to, validated.

Through active listening, we can also reconnect with them at an agreed future time to discuss budgets and therapy provision again. This conversation may proceed along the lines of: 'Given what you have said about how budgets may change for the better in six months' time, and since you have budget responsibilities for the service, could we meet again at the end of the year to catch up about everything?' Just as a therapist creates new client possibilities we can do the same in our conversations with commissioners.

It's important to remember that commissioners (school leaders, hospital managers, social workers, etc.) are also passionate advocates for the people they support. By active listening and creating conversations you allow commissioners to (re)connect with their passion and vitality for the work they do. Co-creating the future possibility of a new therapy service with them, where innovative outcomes for clients/patients may evolve, is a powerful act and the basis of a longer-term partnership.

By bringing active therapeutic-style listening to conversations withcommissioners, therapists are also able to manage expectations, both theirs and the commissioners. The authors' experience of developing therapy work suggests a 10 to 1 ratio of organisations a therapist may need to start talking with to generate a new job or therapy service. With this in mind, 'no' becomes a very normal and to-be-expected part of the journey. It may be helpful for therapists to reflect on the many ways that a client says 'no' and rejects the therapist in a session to see if this ratio is also present at the same level in the therapy room. Our experience suggests that it is.

Through active listening, we can manage the expectations of commissioners, clients and ourselves alike in terms of therapy outcomes. The commissioner may seek to maximise 'bums on seats' within the proposed therapy service. Acknowledging that they have targets to meet and helping them to achieve these realistically and ethically is important. Depending on the referral issues highlighted by commissioners, group work may be more appropriate, and allow more clients to access therapy; however, the therapist should also bring integrity and a knowledge of group therapy approaches that may be suitable to this conversation. Such a discussion may proceed like this:

> I know that ensuring all the students in school can access music therapy is important to you. I'm aware that in Australia Professor Kat McFerran and colleagues [McFerran 2014] are leading the way in specialising in a whole school approach. I'll ask her advice on how we do this and then come back to discuss it with you.

Empathy

To know what others want requires empathy: the ability to understand and share the feelings of others. Empathy is a very human trait, and one that therapists are trained in. Through training, therapists hone their ability to understand their clients and their world (through empathy) without possessing the client's world (through boundaries) (Corey 1991). Empathy makes us aware of and available to others by being able to understand their emotions and circumstances (McLaren 2013). It is a skill that we learn, and it is a social and emotional skill that we are all born with, that helps us to connect to and interact with others (McLaren 2013).

Empathy is currently a hot topic of research in neuroscience, social science and early childhood settings. In a narcissistic world of selfies and Instagram, empathy may not be the first word that springs to mind. Karla McLaren, in her book *The Art of Empathy* (2013), defines empathy as 'a social and emotional skill that helps us feel and understand the emotions, circumstances, intentions, thoughts, and needs of others, such that we can offer sensitive, perceptive, and appropriate communication and support' (p.16).

In our therapeutic work we use empathy all the time. These same skills are vital in the business world on many levels. The first level is that of your client. In a private practice, if you are not empathic to your client's needs they will not return to purchase your services.

Second, if you are not empathic to the needs of commissioners, institutions and communities, you will not offer a service that meets the needs, nor will you understand the emotions that drive the need, or the feelings associated with the needs. To put it bluntly, you won't understand the *why*. Why would people pay for your service in the first place? Once you know this you can think about what you need to do to support them empathically.

Third, you have to understand cash flow in and out of your business, as well as what motivates people to spend it (we have touched on this above). You need to understand the ultimate source of your revenue. Consider government revenue: have you ever stopped and asked yourself who pays for this service? The taxpayer does. Governments are responsible to the taxpayer for public expenditure so you'll need to take into account issues of accountability, compliance and reporting. To overcharge rates to a government-subsidised service shows no empathy to the people who work hard and pay tax in our societies to provide money for services.

When you do not have a guaranteed flow of income, such as government funding, you are more likely to be empathic when considering cash flow and fee structures. This can be very challenging and confronting as there are many complexities at play. As business owners we may have to pay therapists who we employ enough to comply with award or minimum wage levels. In some cases though, pay scales don't exist for creative arts therapies or psychotherapy. This means the pay rate is then set by a tension between what the therapist thinks they are worth, and what the market may bear. In private practice this can be a significant challenge; we need to strike a balance between what the therapist thinks they are worth, what our clients can afford to pay, and what the business needs to charge to cover its costs and generate a profit to remain viable. Overpaying staff sets them up with unrealistic expectations of what the market will bear and makes our profession too expensive for the average person to access. Underpaying sets up the business to fail in the long term. Finding a balance requires empathy. For more detailed information on this and the ethical implications see Chapter 5.

Conclusion

RAILE is a dynamic and non-linear process. RAILE seeks to build the confidence of therapists, to have conversations about service development and the selling of therapy, by building on everyday core clinical skills. Through this process we hope commissioners, and ultimately clients, will benefit by accessing a wide and varied range of therapy services and modalities. We hope also that therapists will begin to realise that standing in the common ground of 'relationship', the often perceived huge gap between therapy and business is merely a footstep or a slight change in perception.

While we acknowledge that for some therapists, a reactive or 'word of mouth' approach to sustaining their caseload is preferred, all therapists use some form of marketing or sales approach to enable potential clients to get in touch. Even in these situations RAILE can enable therapists to feel confident in the often tricky conversations about money or a client's ability to pay, or how expectations of therapy could be communicated in a way that is meaningful to the client, and also ethical and responsible. Everyone wants some certainty about what they will get for their money, regardless of if they are buying a holiday or engaging in therapy.

Go and do it!

We hope these activities below help you to start thinking about your relationship to money within the context of therapy. You should be as honest as you can. You can repeat the activities from time to time to see how your relationship with money might be changing.

Exercise 1: Create a 'money map'

- Take a large sheet of paper and write the word 'money' in the centre. Spend 15 minutes writing down everything that your associate with the word 'money'. Please be as honest as you can, and write down the positive and negative associations you may have. For example, you might write down: wages, greed, holidays, freedom, I love it, having more, rich people, guilt, etc.

- Using all the words on your paper, combine the most salient ones into one sentence that clarifies what money means to you. For example, your sentence may read, 'I love having money and the freedom it gives me, but feel guilty about poor people when I'm on holiday.'

- Next, take this sentence and keep only the *three* most important words, for example 'freedom, guilt, holiday'.

- Then take those three words, and refine down to *two* words, for example 'freedom, guilt'.

- Finally, choose *one* of those words to keep, for example 'freedom'.

This final word can be seen as your current relationship with money. You should try this activity a number of times to see if/how your relationship with money changes over time.

Exercise 2: Fees and charging activity

Write down the three things that make you most uncomfortable about asking for money/charging clients for your therapy services. For example, you may feel that 'Charging people who are sick makes me feel guilty' or 'I hate it when school leaders ask me if I can give them a discounted rate – I always say "Yes" but I want to say "No".'

Doing this activity may help you to uncover some of the fears and conflicting emotions you have about charging money for therapy services. By writing them down, you may start to feel more empowered to think about whether your fears are true or not.

Exercise 3: Improvising with words: 'Yes, and' rather than 'No, but...'

We hope this activity enables you to transfer one of your core clinical skills, improvisation, from your therapy modality (music, drama, play, etc.) into words. We want you to find as much freedom to improvise with your words as you already have within your modality. You'll need to work with a partner for this activity.

- Choose who is the commissioner (A) and who is the therapist (B). The commissioner (A) should come up with a really bizarre or unusual request for therapy services. The therapist (B) should then answer A's request by saying, 'Yes, and...' The Therapist (B) is not allowed to say, 'No, but'.

- An example conversation might go like this:

A: 'I would like music therapy for a large group of students who don't really speak English as a first language, and don't share a language. They also all have behaviour issues. There are about 25 of them. Can you work with them all together, as I want them to use music therapy to make friends and behave better?'

B: 'Yes, and I can see how the behaviour issues you describe and the fact that they don't find it easy to talk with each other might lead to frustration and a lack of friendships in the group. Working with all 25 of them in one go would mean that I would need a member of school staff to help me. Is this possible?'

A: 'I can ask a teaching assistant to help you. So how will you help them? I'm worried it will be chaos in the room, due to their behaviour issues.'

B: 'Yes, and I understand your concern about this. I'm aware that in Germany and Australia there are approaches to working with large groups of children. The German approach is called DrumPower [DrumPower Against Violence 2016]. I'll contact them to ask for their advice and then come back to you with my ideas about how to take this project forward.'

What is important here is that the therapist is able to continue the conversation in an ethical way, which keeps the conversation alive. It is also important to understand what 'Yes, and' actually means.

The 'Yes' is an acknowledgement of the request; it's a way to communicate that the request has been heard and understood. The 'Yes' is non-judgemental, and is neutral to the validity of the request. The 'and' is about the therapist's willingness to remain in the conversation and explore ways in which the request might be answered or met. The 'and' has always got to be rooted in an ethical response and seek to clarify the aims of the request, while looking for an ethical way to proceed.

References

Abad, V. (2003). A time of turmoil: Music therapy interventions for adolescents in a paediatric oncology ward. *Australian Journal of Music Therapy*, 14, 20–37.

Abad, V. (2011). *The effectiveness of a short-term group music therapy intervention for young parents and their children*. Masters Research Thesis, Queensland University of Technology.

Abad, V. and Edwards, J. (2004). Strengthening families: A role for music therapy in contributing to family centred care. *Australian Journal of Music Therapy*, 15, 3–17.

Abad, V. and Thomas, D. (2013). The Economics of Therapy. 39th Australian Music Therapy Association Conference, Sydney, Australia.

Abad, V. and Williams, K. (2006). Early intervention music therapy for adolescent mothers and their children. *British Journal of Music Therapy*, 20, 31–38.

Abad, V. and Williams, K. (2007). Early intervention music therapy: Reporting on a 3-year project to address needs with at-risk families. *Music Therapy Perspectives*, 25, 1, 52–58.

American Psychological Association (2016). *What is resilience?* PsychCentral. Retrieved from http://psychcentral.com/lib/what-is-resilience on 25 November 2016.

Chaplin, W.F., Phillips, J.B., Brown, N., Clanton, R. and Stein, J.L. (2000) Handshaking, gender, personality, and first impressions. *Journal of Personality and Social Psychology*, 79, 1, 110–117.

Corey, G. (1991). *Theory and Practice of Counseling and Psychotherapy (4th Edition)*. Belmont, CA: Brooks/Cole Publishing Co.

Creighton, A., Atherton, M. and Kitamura, C. (2013). Singing play songs and lullabies: Investigating the subjective contributions to maternal attachment constructs. *Australian Journal of Music Therapy*, 24, 17–44.

Docherty, S.L., Robb, S.L., Phillips-Salimi, C., Cherven, B., Stegenga, K., Hendricks-Ferguson, V. *et al.* (2013). Parental perspectives on the behavioural health intervention for music adolescent/young adult resilience during cancer treatment: Report from the children's oncology group. *Journal of Adolescent Health*, 52, 2, 170.

Donnelly, L. (2015). Handshake strength 'could predict' heart attack risk. *The Lancet*, 14 May. Retrieved at www.telegraph.co.uk/journalists/laura-donnelly/11603129/Handshake-strength-could-predict-heart-attack-risk.html on 25 November 2016.

DrumPower Against Violence. (2016). *Home Page*. Retrieved at www.trommelpower-gegen-gewalt.de/en on 16 January 2017.

Edwards, J. (2011). Music therapy and parent-infant bonding. In J. Edwards (ed.), *Music Therapy and Parent–Infant Bonding* (pp.5–21). Oxford: Oxford University Press.

Edwards, J. and Abad, V. (2016). Music therapy and parent–infant programmes. In J. Edwards (ed.), *The Oxford Handbook of Music Therapy* (pp.135–157). Oxford: Oxford University Press.

Malloch, S. and Trevarthen, C. (2009). Musicality: Communicating the vitality and interests of life. In S. Malloch and C. Trevarthen (eds), *Communicative Musicality: Exploring the Basis of Human Companionship* (pp.1–11). Oxford: Oxford University Press.

Masten, A.S. (2001). Ordinary magic: Resilience processes in development. *American Psychologist*, 56, 3, 227–238.

Masten, A.S. (2011). Resilience in children threatened by extreme adversity: Frameworks for research, practice, and translational synergy. *Development and Psychopathology*, 23, 2, 493–506.

McFerran, K.S. (2014). Music therapy in the schools. In B. Wheeler (ed.), *Music Therapy Handbook* (pp.328–338). New York: Guildford Press.

McLaren, K. (2013). *The Art of Empathy*. Boulder, CO: Sounds True.

Nicholson, J.M., Berthelsen, D., Abad, V., Williams, K. and Bradley, J. (2008). Impact of music therapy to promote positive parenting and child development. *Journal of Health Psychology*, 13, 2, 226–238.

Oldfield, A. (2011). Parents' perceptions of being in music therapy sessions with their children: What is our role as music therapists with parents? In J. Edwards (ed.), *Music Therapy and Parent–Infant Bonding* (pp.58–72). Oxford: Oxford University Press.

Pasiali, V. (2010). *Family-based music therapy: Fostering child resilience and promoting parental self-efficacy through shared musical experiences*. PhD thesis, Michigan State University.

Pink, D. (2014). *To Sell is Human*. Edinburgh: Canongate Books Ltd.

Queensland University of Technology (2016). *Personal Transferable Skills*. Retrieved from www.careers.qut.edu.au/student/resource/transferable.pdf on 25 November 2016.

Robb, S.L., Burns, D.S., Stegenga, K.A., Haut, P.R., Monahan, P.O., Meza, J. *et al.* (2014). Randomized clinical trial of therapeutic music video intervention for resilience outcomes in adolescents/young adults undergoing hematopoietic stem cell transplant: A report from the Children's Oncology Group. *Cancer* 120, 6, 909–917.

Ruksenas, J. (2013). *Singing as Resilience: The Missing Link in Education?* International Congress of Voice Teachers, Brisbane, Australia.

Stern, D. (2000). *The Interpersonal World of the Infant*. New York: Basic Books.

Vocabulary.com (n.d.) *Improvisation*. Retrieved from www.vocabulary.com/dictionary/improvisation on 26 November 2016.

Wigram, T. (2004). *Improvisation: Methods and Techniques for Music Therapy Clinicians, Educators and Students*. London: Jessica Kingsley Publishers.

Willis, J. and Todorov, A. (2006). First impressions: Making up your mind after 100ms exposure to a face. *Psychological Science* 17, 1, 592–598.

Winnicott, D.W. (1987 [1952]). Letter to Roger Money-Kyrle, 27th November. In *The Spontaneous Gesture: Selected Letters of D.W. Winnicott* (pp.38–43). London: Karnac Books.

Winsler, A., Ducenne, L. and Koury, A. (2011). Singing one's way to self-regulation: The role of early music and movement curricula and private speech. *Early Education and Development*, 22, 274–304.

CHAPTER 4

For What It's Worth...
Determining the Value of Music Therapy - An Example from Austria
Monika Geretsegger, Elena Fitzthum and Thomas Stegemann

Introduction

Although sharing the profession of music therapists, we as authors of this chapter have different training backgrounds, secondary professions and additional honorary functions that are all related to different perspectives on the economics of therapy. We would like to share and integrate these views and experiences using the example of Austria. In Austria, arts therapies such as music therapy, art therapy and drama therapy are nowadays represented in various areas of health care and pedagogical settings. This includes arts therapists working in hospitals, care facilities, rehabilitation centres, schools or private practices.

In this chapter we will use music therapy as a paradigm to explore how the value of arts in therapy might be determined within an Austrian context. This is because music therapy has the longest history of academic training and is comparatively well established in many clinical institutions.

This chapter will provide an overview of the Austrian health care system, including a background on the historical development of music therapy within it, followed by information about music therapy training and how it feeds into the profession and its perceived value. We recognise that other arts therapies may experience similar issues and therefore aim to provide information that addresses the questions of value for all arts therapies through a music therapy paradigm.

As a result of the continuing process of professionalisation of music therapy, the Music Therapists Act came into effect in 2009

(Mössler 2008a; *Musiktherapiegesetz* 2016). In the first place, it serves to ensure an obligatory professional standard, thus protecting the client's/patient's rights and safety. It encompasses the regulation of framework conditions of the music therapy training as well as music therapists' legal obligations and responsibilities. The law does not include any regulations or guidelines concerning financial aspects and fees. Some might think that a specific law for music therapy would directly impact the funding of music therapy, but it is important to note that such a regulation is necessary, although not sufficient for solving questions about financing. While costs for music therapy are often covered in institutional contexts in Austria, it is still the clients themselves who need to pay the fees incurred for music therapy in private practice.

Background
Health care system in Austria
When talking about economic aspects of arts therapies in general, and music therapy in particular, it is crucial to consider the circumstances of a country´s health care system, where therapists provide their services, and where they are both in cooperation and in competition with other health care providers.

Austria, located in central Europe, has approximately 8.5 million inhabitants. With a gross domestic product (GDP) of €300.7 billion in 2011, which is equivalent to €35, 710 per capita, Austria is one of the richest countries in the world; in 2011, 10.8 per cent of the GDP was spent on health, corresponding to about €3848 per capita (Austrian Federal Ministry of Health 2013).

The Austrian social and health care system is primarily based on the principle of compulsory social insurance. It is mainly financed through a combination of income-based social insurance contributions, public income generated through taxes, and private payments in the form of direct and indirect co-payments. Access to services is regulated by law, thus offering a large number of benefits to all insured people, that is, 99.9 per cent of the population (Austrian Federal Ministry of Health 2013). This includes access to a variety of services, for example primary health care, emergency care, specialised in-patient and outpatient care, maternity services, health technology such as X-ray and laboratory tests, dental services and psychotherapy, and also physiotherapy, occupational therapy, speech therapy, curative massage and similar therapies provided by health professionals other than physicians.

This means that practically all Austrian inhabitants, independent of their income, age, sex or origin, are guaranteed free access to health care services, in terms of primary care. Psychotherapy, for example, is financed by co-payment (statutory insurance compensation per session: €21.80). Although music therapy is a health care profession which is regulated by a federal law (see details below), until now it has only been financed within institutional services (in-patient care), and not in outpatient care.

Private health care expenditure primarily consists of household out-of-pocket payments and expenditure by private insurance companies. According to the latest data from Statistics Austria (2015), these health care costs grew from €2574 million in 1990 to €7277 million in 2013, which is equivalent to an average annual growth rate of 4.6 per cent. Outpatient care, with a share of 36.4 per cent, was the largest expenditure category of private households and private insurance enterprises. This development, which is similar to the situation in other European countries (Austrian Federal Ministry of Health 2013), shows that the private health care sector, in particular concerning out-of-pocket payments, represents an enormous growth market.

In addition, current developments in health care economy increasingly prioritise novel approaches in public health care due to increasing cost pressure. This is demonstrated in the following quote by the Austrian Federal Minister of Health and Women's Affairs, Sabine Oberhauser: 'It is particularly important to me that health care policy is not just about repair-based medicine, but about promoting and preserving people's health and the prevention of illness' (Oberhauser 2016).

Through its holistic approach, music therapy might have something to contribute to a paradigm shift in public health care, which seems to be necessary to guarantee today's high standard of health care services, affordable for everyone, for future times.

Music therapy in the Austrian health care system

The beginnings of music therapy in Austria date back to the late 1950s, making Austria one of the pioneering countries for music therapy in Europe (Gold 2003; Halmer-Stein *et al.* 1993). Music therapy in Austria was embedded in clinical settings from the very beginning: the first music therapy positions and internships were located in the fields of psychiatry and care for people with special needs, followed by the area of psychosomatics (Mössler 2011).

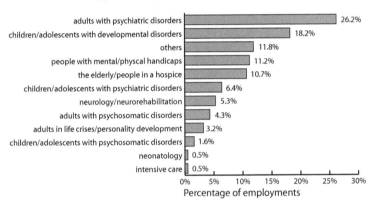

THE CURRENT SITUATION:
Music therapy as a recognised health profession in Austria

Figure 4.1 Distribution of music therapy employments in Austria across different areas of work; data taken from a survey conducted in 2011, *n* = 131 (adapted from Geretsegger *et al.* 2012)

Today, music therapy is practised in many sectors of the health care system in Austria. In the latest survey conducted by the Austrian Association of Music Therapists (Geretsegger, Böhm-Öppinger & Schmidtmayr 2012), we found that adult mental health is by far the largest field of work, comprising 30.5 per cent of all music therapy employments in Austria when adults with psychiatric and psychosomatic disorders are taken together; 24.6 per cent of all music therapy employments in Austria are in the treatment of children and adolescents with developmental disorders, behavioural problems and psychiatric disorders. Other large client groups for music therapists in Austria are people with mental and/or physical handicaps (11.2%) and the elderly/people in hospices (10.7%).

Figure 4.1 gives an overview of the employment percentages for these and other areas of work.

More than a quarter (26.8%) of all Austrian music therapy employments can be found in hospitals, followed by the categories private practice (22.3%) and outpatient clinic (15.0%); see Figure 4.2.

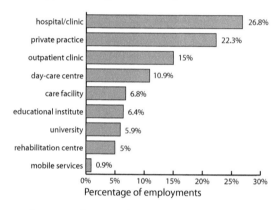

THE CURRENT SITUATION:
Music therapy as a recognised health profession in Austria

Figure 4.2 Distribution of music therapy employments in Austria in relation to types of workplace; data taken from a 2011 survey, n = 131 (adapted from Geretsegger *et al.* 2012)

Although almost one quarter of all Austrian music therapy positions are in private practice (Geretsegger *et al.* 2012), the number of patients treated in outpatient care is still quite small, and negligible in comparison to the music therapy services provided in institutions like psychiatric hospitals. This is primarily due to the fact that music therapy patients in outpatient care have to bear the costs by themselves without being entitled to receive refunds through health insurance.

According to recommendations by the Austrian Association of Music Therapists (2015), fees for music therapy in private practice should not be below a minimum of €55 for one-on-one sessions in private practice, and not below €100 for sessions in a group setting.

The price level for psychotherapy in Austria is slightly different: in private practice, costs typically range from €70 to 150 for one-on-one sessions, with a regular insurance reimbursement rate of €21.80 (Hofbauer 2015). Costs for occupational therapy, physiotherapy, and speech and language therapy can be fully reimbursed (provided an appropriate indication is present), but there are often waiting lists of a couple of months, particularly for children. In contrast, art therapy is not regulated by law in Austria. Hence, the profession is not protected, and its services cannot be funded by the public health sector, so that all costs for art therapy usually need to be paid by clients themselves.

The Austrian Music Therapists Act

The Music Therapists Act came into effect on 1 July 2009, after a decades-long process of efforts and negotiations to gain state recognition, and a unanimous parliamentary vote in June 2008 (Mössler 2008a). Since then, music therapy is one of the legally regulated health professions in Austria, making the country one of the few in the world where the music therapy profession is officially recognised. The Music Therapists Act defines two types of professional qualification: music therapists who are entitled to work independently (based on a bachelor's plus master's qualification in music therapy), and those who work with shared responsibility (based on a bachelor's qualification in music therapy). Music therapists in Austria have to fulfil certain criteria (regarding training, occupational duties, etc.) to be registered in the official Music Therapists list run by the Ministry of Health. At the time of writing this chapter (May 2016), 346 music therapists are listed therein, 36 of them as working with shared responsibility (cf. the Music Therapists list at Austrian Federal Ministry of Health and Women's Affairs n.d.). For a summary of key contents and characteristics of the Austrian Music Therapists Act, see Mössler (2008a).

In the first place, the Music Therapists Act serves to define music therapy as a profession within the Austrian health care system, including rights and obligations as well as a code of conduct for music therapists. In addition, it provides quality assurance by setting professional standards in music therapy training, music therapy practice, and continuing professional development. Thus, the Music

Therapists Act assures a certain level of qualification which primarily serves to protect patients and clients who are receiving music therapy. Moreover, it is hoped that recognition as a legally regulated health profession will open new doors concerning negotiations about music therapy funding with health care providers and health insurers. This represents a very relevant issue, as the Music Therapists Act as such has nothing to do with financial affairs. Therefore, recognition as a legally regulated health profession might prove helpful in claiming adequate salaries for music therapists, and for a (co-)funding of music therapy by health care insurances, but neither can be taken for granted. In fact, it cannot be ruled out that hospitals might be tempted to employ music therapists with a lower degree only, particularly in times of economic crisis. In the worst case, this might lead to a general decrease in music therapy salaries.

Music therapy training

The beginnings of an academic music therapy education in Austria date back to the year 1959, when the first training course was established at what was then the Vienna Academy of Music (today's University of Music and Performing Arts Vienna). It was founded and headed by the Austrian violinist Editha Koffer-Ullrich. Her successor, Alfred Schmölz, a former piano teacher, was influential in subsequently shaping the course and pioneering what is now called the 'Viennese School of Music Therapy' (Mössler 2011).

Today there are three training courses, located in Graz, Krems and Vienna. These courses work together as collaborators rather than competitors in a panel called 'ÖMAK – Österreichische Musiktherapie-AusbildungsleiterInnenkonferenz' (Austrian Music Therapy Education Conference) to promote continuing cooperation and exchange between the three institutes regarding issues in education, research and practice. The resulting signal effect of academic training courses acting in concert – instead of being trapped in competitive battle – cannot be overestimated. Despite all diversity, speaking with one voice, and concerted actions of both academic training courses and professional associations, is an indispensable prerequisite for achieving common goals concerning legal regulations (see the section 'The Austrian Music Therapists Act' above) and funding for our profession.

When looking at today's four-year, full-time music therapy training course in Vienna, there is an extensive entrance exam consisting of three days of testing and evaluating the musical and personal competencies of the candidates. At the end of the assessment procedure, only ten out of about 60 to 80 applicants can be enrolled. The restriction of admission in Vienna is mainly due to limited capacities for one-on-one tuition (main music instrument/vocals) and to limited clinical internship positions, which are fully integrated in the curriculum (minimum of 765 hours practical training, including clinical supervision and complementary medical seminars). It is a central tenet of the Viennese training course that both individual music therapy self-experience, and music therapy self-experience in a group are essential and obligatory parts of the curriculum, adding up to 270 hours in three years. This is in line with what has been described as a specific principle of a self-experience-based music therapy orientation by Bonde (2015), 'that a music therapist must go through a personal MT process in order to establish a well-grounded professional identity' (p.173). Of course, the expenses for one-on-one tuition and self-experience are quite high, and in many training programmes, those elements are therefore not included in tuition fees. From a psychodynamically as well as a humanistically informed understanding of music therapy, these personal and professional skills can only be achieved through continuing music therapy self-experience – whatever the costs!

Talking about money: fees for music therapy courses in Europe vary significantly. As an example, comparing the tuition fees of only the state-approved music therapy training courses of the German-speaking countries reveals that the total costs for a master's degree may range between some €150 and more than €30,000 (Stegemann et al. 2013). Although all Austrian universities have been charging tuition fees since the summer semester of 2013, there are exemptions from payment for citizens of EU member states. Thus, in fact, the vast majority of students have to pay only the membership fee for the Austrian student self-administration, which is currently €18.70 per semester. When looking at training courses in Europe, total costs for a master's degree range from none (in some Scandinavian countries) to almost €40,000 for international students in the UK (Stegemann et al. 2016).

Still, in comparison to psychotherapy training courses in Austria (with an average of total cost of more than €70,000; cf. bestNET Information-Service 2016), music therapy training courses are quite affordable. Apparently, psychotherapy candidates are willing to pay more than twice as much for their degree, often accepting economic strains for many years before the investment pays off. At least – due to higher wage levels (cf. the section 'Music therapy in the Austrian health care system' above) and possibly to better reputation – it seems to be worth the effort. This makes a huge difference to the situation of music therapists, who usually have to have another string to their bow (besides a half-time employment as music therapist) to earn a living. As a consequence, there is the imminent danger that due to economic pressure those responsible for music therapy training courses might be tempted to reduce tuition fees by excluding cost-intensive courses as obligatory elements of their curriculum (e.g. individual self-experience). Thus, their programme would become more affordable for candidates and more competitive in comparison to other training courses. It goes without saying that such tendencies might lead to a vicious circle, resulting in decreasing quality standards in education which might in turn entail lower salaries, and so on. Further, it may have adverse consequences for the self-conception and the self-image of a music therapist, which will be addressed in the next section of this chapter.

The value of music therapy from various perspectives

If seeking to specify the value of music therapy, different contexts may be taken into account (see Figure 4.3).

Even though some of the perspectives elaborated on below may seem quite general, we believe that reflecting on several of these levels will help to better determine one's own stance towards the value of music therapy. We consider this to be particularly relevant for therapists in early stages of their professional careers, as well as for colleagues working in countries where music therapy is less established as yet, or still in a pioneer status.

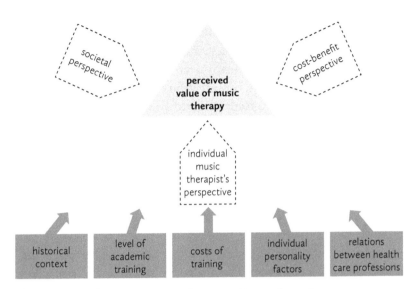

Figure 4.3 Various contexts and perspectives relevant to the perceived value of music therapy

First, from a *societal perspective*, one can explore how music therapy contributes to a society's culture. This includes questions about the value of joint musical experiences, such as making music together and listening to music, impacting, for instance, on proportions of music education in school curricula, public funding for music events, or using music as a means of promoting relationships within communities.

Socio-cultural aspects of music therapy and possible interconnections with societal changes and government policies have been explored by various authors (e.g. Bunt & Stige 2014). For example, a vision of music therapy as a socially engaged practice that might contribute to a more just society with equal access to music has been described by Even Ruud (1980), and the potential of musical participation to promote social inclusion has been pointed out particularly in the context of community music therapy (Stige & Aarø 2012).

Societal perspectives on music therapy may also be linked to the remarkable role that music might have played as a crucial factor in the evolution of humans and their brains, and in the development of spoken language (Cross 2009; Fitch 2012; Mithen 2009). This notion has been elaborated on, and expanded by, Stefan Koelsch in his concept called the 'seven Cs' (Koelsch & Stegemann 2012).

The 'seven Cs' constitute different areas of social activities that are proposed to be promoted and facilitated through joint music-making (contact, social cognition, co-pathy – referring to the social function of empathy – communication, coordination of actions, cooperation and social cohesion). This concept seeks to combine a neurobiological and a socio-psychological approach, which may offer a suitable theoretical framework to determine and to underpin the impact of music on society, and the role that can be assigned to music therapy.

Additionally, music therapy as a health profession may be more or less well known among the public, and awareness about music therapy's potential is certainly connected with attributions of higher or lower value.

Second, the value of music therapy may be seen from a *cost–benefit* perspective: to what extent does music therapy help achieve specified goals, for example in the treatment of illnesses and disorders, in relation to its costs? There is still hardly any research into the cost-effectiveness of music therapy comparing it with other forms of treatment in various areas. However, several studies have shown that music therapy is an effective treatment and thus represents a value on its own, for instance for people with serious mental health disorders (Gold *et al.* 2009), people with autism spectrum disorder (Geretsegger *et al.* 2014), or people with dementia (Ridder *et al.* 2013). Especially in areas where other treatments are not (yet) feasible, as in people with low motivation to attend any kind of therapy (Gold *et al.* 2013), or people with impaired language abilities, music therapy can serve as a means to promote health, and sometimes to reduce medication or other costly interventions, thus lowering consequential expenses for treatment, and general economic costs.

Third, from the *individual perspective* of a music therapist setting up a private practice, questions about the value of music therapy have immediate importance in the process of *setting fees* for therapy services that are feasible both for clients/patients and the therapist themselves. Providing health care for clients/patients, particularly as an arts therapist in private practice, may be an area of conflicting economic priorities as service users are often socially disadvantaged, while the therapist still needs to make a living from being a health care professional (cf. Dileo 2000).

The two perspectives described above, societal value and cost-effectiveness of music therapy, may also be influential in the development of one´s identity as a therapist/health care provider. In further consequence, such self-conceptions may become modifiers within the third context, setting therapy fees for various groups of clients. In the following section, we will discuss additional factors, motives and rationales that may – consciously or unconsciously – influence expectations and decisions about the amount of money due for one's therapy services.

Factors, motives and rationales that influence our expectations and decisions about the value of arts therapies

Understanding how historical context impacts the perception of current value

As described above, the history of music therapy in Austria goes back several decades – longer than in most European countries. In the early days of music therapy in the USA and in several European countries, mainly women were working as music therapists – usually on a voluntary basis without being paid. These volunteers usually were upper-class women – who else, during the first half of the 20th century, would have had the opportunity to study music without the pressure of making a living out of it? Many of them were piano teachers who strove for a chance to actively participate in work life using their musical skills (cf. Fitzthum 2003). Back then, most men simply could not afford to engage in this type of voluntary occupation, as they usually were expected to feed a family. As pioneers of music therapy in Austria, Albertine Wesecky and Ilse Castelliz worked on a voluntary basis in a hospital for a long time before they received remuneration for teaching at the Vienna Academy of Music. Both of them played a major role in building up music therapy in a clinical setting; they started to publish their work, and to train the 'second generation' of music therapists in Austria (Fitzthum 2003). According to Mössler's description of the distinct stages of development of the Viennese School of Music Therapy (2008b), it would be fair to speak of a phase of transition which is taking place right now: the third generation of music therapists are taking over from the second generation to train the next generation. This close interaction and integration of different generations of music therapists who meet and cooperate in several different areas (such as practical work, education and advocacy) has an enormous impact on the development of the profession: not only does it help develop a feeling of coherence within this group, based on a long tradition and shared history, but it also provides a secure base from which one's professional identity as a music therapist can be established. This facilitates the music therapist's individual work and the public's perception of music therapy as a profession.

Understanding how the level of academic training impacts the perception of value

Over the past decades, training programmes for music therapy in many European countries have moved from privately run or non-academic courses to full study programmes at universities. In Austria, the former two-year 'Sonderlehrgang für Musikheilkunde' (Special Training Programme for Music Medical Science, established in 1959) at the Academy of Music turned into a 'Lehrgang Musiktherapie' (Music Therapy Training Programme) in 1970, then further into a six-semester course ('Kurzstudium', Short Study Programme) in 1992. In 2003, the music therapy programme was turned into an eight-semester, full academic training course with a master's-equivalent degree at what was by then the University of Music and Performing Arts, Vienna (MDW). New university regulations introduced in 2002 permitted the establishment of PhD-level training in music therapy which eventually started at the MDW in October 2013.

The fact that music therapy has turned into an academic discipline undoubtedly served the profession well in Austria, as it provided a favourable foundation for becoming a legally recognised health care profession. Today, the regulation of the profession by the Austrian Music Therapists Act specifies that music therapists must at least hold a bachelor's degree in music therapy to practise the profession with 'shared responsibility', and – in addition to a music therapy bachelor's degree – a master's degree (or equivalent) for practising with 'sole responsibility'. However, this process of increasing the level of academic training along with the introduction of the three-level system of university education following the Bologna reforms (aiming to facilitate students' mobility by introducing specified criteria for bachelor's, master's and doctoral degrees) have also brought about difficulties regarding adequate remuneration: the two types of professional occupation in Austria (shared vs. sole responsibility with bachelor's vs. master's degrees) would suggest a two-tier salary structure for music therapists, and salaries in the range of other academic professions in health care. Although in recent times, and with the rising reputation of music therapy as a profession, salaries at some clinical institutions have been higher than in earlier times, there is a risk that wages might be downgraded from corresponding to a master's degree to the bachelor's level. This is already the case in some Austrian hospitals where, after the implementation of the Music Therapists Act, and due to cost-cutting measures following budget cutbacks, new employees – regardless of whether or not they hold a master's degree in music therapy – are now hired at a salary that corresponds to a bachelor qualification, as employers deem this level sufficient for this type of work within clinical institutions.

Understanding that high-quality training costs money

In Austria, the scope of training standards is defined in the Music Therapists Act. This includes high levels of musical proficiency and personal as well as professional competencies, clinical internships, supervision, and theoretical knowledge of music therapy and neighbouring disciplines. All this costs a lot of money, so both the academic level and the quality of music therapy education do not come for free. In times of budget cuts, financial limitations often lead to circumstances where core elements of music therapy training programmes (such as costly one-on-one courses) are jeopardised. However, in view of the considerable challenges that therapists face in their daily clinical practice, economic cuts that lead to reduced-quality standards in training would be negligent both towards patients/clients and therapists.

It is important to note that training programmes that are financed by students' fees only are usually working under conditions different from those that are mainly government-financed (as is the case for state-run programmes in some countries). Particularly in newly established programmes, especially in Eastern and Southern Europe, the target number of students can only be achieved if expenses for training are kept at a low level.

Understanding how individual personality factors impact the perception of value

It is quite a safe assumption that the core interests of people who consider becoming arts therapists, and music therapists in particular, are not primarily in making lots of money through their profession. Often, these are people who want to help others, and often, they have a strong sense of empathy – a trait that can become some sort of a hindrance when, after their studies, they need to enforce their salary expectations.

Another difficulty for graduates might lie in a common phenomenon that has been described as the 'impostor phenomenon' (Huffstutler & Varnell 2006) – a potential psychological barrier in people who are objectively competent but feel the opposite, and therefore fear being unmasked. Such a dilemma – feeling like a greenhorn while having a first-class education as a health care specialist – might function as an additional obstacle in receiving adequate remuneration for one's services. Especially when confronted with the complexity of clinical challenges for the first time (after experiences in the rather 'protected' area of clinical internships during studies), the self-esteem, motivation and stamina necessary for successful salary negotiations are often low.

Understanding how relationships and power relations between various health care professions impact the perception of value

Both young professionals and experienced music therapists are only too familiar with situations where they not only need to negotiate salaries and justify fees, but need to explain what it is they are actually doing, and for what purpose – quite different from other, more established health care professions. While music therapy has nowadays grown out of its pioneer status in many European countries, it is still possible that a music therapist, in particular if working in rural areas, is involuntarily thrown back to a pioneer role in their profession. Also in Austria, especially outside the metropolitan area of Vienna, where music therapy has evolved close to universities and hospitals, the discrepancy between a music therapist's own professional self-concept on the one hand, including a wealth of acquired knowledge, personal competency and clinical skills, and the public perception of the profession on the other hand, can be considerable. Local advocacy work focused on regional areas, both by individual therapists and by network initiatives and professional associations, is often needed to increase public awareness of the music therapy profession, and also increase the awareness of other health professions and decision-makers in the health care system.

Another approach to improving the perception of arts therapies in relation to other professions in health care is to specifically describe the competencies of arts therapists in official documents, similar to comparable documents for other health care professions. In addition to the professional requirements that are already defined in the Austrian Music Therapists Act, more detailed guidelines describing specific competencies which music therapy students need to acquire by the end of their studies are currently being developed by the Austrian Ministry of Health together with representatives of training courses and professional associations. Thus, both the comprehensibility and the visibility of music therapy in the context of the health care system are expected to improve further, which can serve as an important step in increasing the profession's value, especially considering power relations between professions that may hitherto have been perceived as asymmetrical (i.e. between larger and more established professions such as physicians and psychologists, and smaller and younger professions such as music or art therapists).

Conclusion

Working in arts therapies raises specific circumstances that set it apart from other ways of making a living, especially when working in the health care sector, treating people with somatic and/or mental disorders and illnesses.

This chapter has outlined the development and current situation of music therapy in Austria to provide a framework for exploring and discussing some of the pertinent issues that impact on how music therapy is perceived and valued. Music therapy was used as an example, as legal regulations for the profession exist, while at the same time, fundamental problems concerning (public) funding of music therapy persist (also cf. Böhm-Öppinger 2015). We have further explored how historical factors and personal as well as professional contexts may contribute to developing a profession's and an individual therapist's sense of self-esteem and societal value, and how this influences the perception of value. The socio-cultural aspects of music and cost–benefit considerations, the profession's history, the level of academic training, its quality standards and costs, individual personality factors, and power relations between health care professions all interact in the development of identity, and identity impacts our perception of what our work is worth.

Through this illustration of complex processes influencing the value of music therapy, we hope that readers will feel encouraged to reflect on their own stance towards the value of music therapy (and other arts therapies), including considerations about relevant factors that influence and modify their personal view. This might also help strengthen a therapist's position when negotiating and justifying remuneration for therapy services with clients, employers, politicians and authorities. Nevertheless, there will often be a mismatch between therapists' perceptions of the value of their work and their professional services and the rewards they will receive in terms of recognition and financial compensation. Such an imbalance, not uncommon in health care professions, stands out even more if compared to typical salaries in other fields of work such as, say, the financial sector, or the entertainment industry. At the end of the day, these issues cannot be solved by individual therapists, or health care professions alone, but are strongly connected to ethical and political questions about what a society is willing to invest to achieve certain prioritised goals.

To quote a pioneer of music therapy, Mary Priestley begins her book *Music Therapy in Action* (1975) with a chapter titled 'What is music therapy?', and the very brief answer is that she views it as more than a profession, but scarcely as a living. Today, 40 years later, it sometimes appears that not too much has changed since then. In a survey about music therapy in child and adolescent psychiatry, conducted in Germany (Stegemann *et al.* 2008), we found music therapists were above average regarding their job satisfaction, although their salaries were sub-standard compared to other health care professionals holding an academic degree. These results might be interpreted as showing that the participants of the study were highly identified with their profession as a music therapist, despite working conditions in need of improvement (besides the salary, this often refers to working space available, or integration into the team on the ward).

Hence for individual music therapists, we consider it important that they venture to take a step that took place some 30 years ago in psychotherapy; it can be summarised in the words 'from confession to profession' – the subtitle of a classic book on psychotherapy research (Grawe, Donati & Bernauer 1994). The time has come to overcome helper syndrome and inferiority complex, and to appreciate one's own value. Interestingly, this might correlate with the amount of time and money one has spent on one's training, personal development and future career as a music therapist. To be confident about one's own profession (including the specific skills only music therapists have, as well as knowledge about limitations of the method) might help to make the step from confession ('It's such a lovely work we do') to profession ('It's necessary to treat this person with music therapy, because A, B and C'). Thus, music therapists would be less prone to suffer from the 'impostor phenomenon' of feeling like a greenhorn while having a first-class education as a health care specialist.

In summary, we would like to emphasise that the value of music therapy, as it is perceived by music therapists themselves, by patients and by society, is highly dependent on the continuing development of standards in research and training, and on the communication of these achievements both within our community and in public.

Go and do it!

We propose that it is most conducive to successfully determining the value of music therapy (e.g. when setting fees for one's services, when discussing one's salary as a therapist, or when negotiating public funding contributions for therapy) if therapists are primarily guided by their professional ethos. With this in mind, and based on our considerations above, we would like to present the following reflective exercises for readers – whether involved in training programmes or professional organisations, individual therapists or students, or others.

Exercise 1: Essentials of a training programme

What would you say are the training constituents that an arts therapy training programme should make sure to preserve as an obligatory part of its curriculum, even in times of austerity measures? Consider the principles that are central to your orientation(s), and how they might be endangered by financial constraints or the temptation of reducing costs by removing costly components due to economic considerations. How would you balance the trade-offs between operating economically and retaining quality, considering the demand for profitability widespread in today's societies and therefore also in the education and health care sectors?

Exercise 2: The role of professional organisations

What do you expect from a professional arts therapy organisation in terms of contributing towards efforts to achieve a solid economic foundation for the profession, and an adequate level of salaries? What roles, respectively, would you say that the following areas of activities play in this process?

- Advocacy work in the general public.

- Cooperation with public bodies.

- Negotiations with authorities and health insurances; conducting surveys about numbers of therapists working in different fields of practice or geographical distribution of services.

- Maintaining, and regularly updating, information about research into arts therapies applied in various fields to document an intervention's efficacy and efficiency.

- Providing continuing professional development opportunities and information material concerning economic aspects of working as a therapist (such as 'How to set up a private practice').

- Regularly following, and observing critical dates regarding legal amendments in, federal and regional legislation and health insurance specifications regarding possible refunds for therapy services to ensure that therapy services are adequately and appropriately classified within existing regulations.

Exercise 3: Profitable collaboration between professions

In your own professional practice, how do you go about finding a balance between cooperation and delimitation in relation to other health care professions? What are your profession's specific contributions to health care, and what possibilities are there for profitable collaboration between professions?

References

Austrian Association of Music Therapists (2015). *Honorarempfehlungen* [Fee recommendations]. Unpublished document. Vienna: Austrian Association of Music Therapists.

Austrian Federal Ministry of Health (2013). *The Austrian Health Care System*. Vienna: BMG. Retrieved from www.bmgf.gv.at/cms/home/attachments/3/4/4/CH1066/CMS1291414949078/austrian_health_care_key_facts_2013.pdf on 15 May 2016.

Austrian Federal Ministry of Health and Women's Affairs (n.d.) *MusiktherapeutInnenliste – Suche*. Retrieved from http://musiktherapie.ehealth.gv.at on 3 December 2016.

bestNET Information-Service (2016). Psychotherapie-Ausbildung [Psychotherapy training]. Vienna: bestNET Information-Service. Retrieved from www.psyonline.at/contents/304 on 15 May 2016.

Bonde, L.O. (2015). The current state of music therapy theory? *Nordic Journal of Music Therapy*, 24, 167–175.

Böhm-Öppinger, S. (2015). Austria – Country report on professional recognition of music therapy. *Approaches: Music Therapy & Special Music Education*, 7 (special issue), 133–134.

Bunt, L. and Stige, B. (2014). *Music Therapy: An Art Beyond Words* (2nd edition). London: Routledge.

Cross, I. (2009). The Nature of Music and its Evolution. In S. Hallam, I. Cross and M. Thaut (eds), *Oxford Handbook of Music Psychology* (pp.3–17). Oxford: Oxford University Press.

Dileo, C. (2000). *Ethical Thinking in Music Therapy*. Cherry Hill, NJ: Jeffrey Books.

Fitch, W.T. (2012). The Biology and Evolution of Rhythm: Unravelling a Paradox. In P. Rebuschat, M. Rohmeier, J.A. Hawkins and I. Cross (eds), *Language and Music as Cognitive Systems* (pp.63–88). Oxford: Oxford University Press.

Fitzthum, E. (2003). *Wiener Beiträge zur Musiktherapie, Band 5: Von den Reformbewegungen zur Musiktherapie. Die Brückenfunktion der Vally Weigl* [Viennese contributions to music therapy, Vol. 5: From reform movements to music therapy. The bridging function of Vally Weigl]. Vienna: Edition Praesens.

Geretsegger, M., Böhm-Öppinger, S. and Schmidtmayr, B. (2012). *Zur beruflichen Situation von MusiktherapeutInnen in Österreich – Ergebnisse einer Erhebung* [On the occupational situation of music therapists in Austria – findings from a survey]. Unpublished report. Vienna: Österreichischer Berufsverband der MusiktherapeutInnen.

Geretsegger, M., Elefant, C., Mössler, K.A. and Gold, C. (2014). Music therapy for people with autism spectrum disorder. *Cochrane Database of Systematic Reviews*, 6. doi: 10.1002/14651858.CD004381.pub3

Gold, C. (2003). *Music therapy in Austria*. Voices Resources. Retrieved from https://voices.no/community/?q=country-of-the-month/2003-music-therapy-austria on 15 May 2016.

Gold, C., Mössler, K., Grocke, D., Heldal, T.O., Tjelmsland, L., Aarre, T. *et al.* (2013). Individual music therapy for mental health care clients with low therapy motivation: Multicentre randomised controlled trial. *Psychotherapy and Psychosomatics*, 82, 319–331.

Gold, C., Solli, H.P., Krüger, V. and Lie, S.A. (2009). Dose–response relationship in music therapy for people with serious mental disorders: Systematic review and meta-analysis. *Clinical Psychology Review*, 29, 193–207.

Grawe, K., Donati, R. and Bernauer, F. (1994). *Psychotherapie im Wandel – Von der Konfession zur Profession* [Psychotherapy in transition – from confession to profession] (3rd edition). Göttingen: Hogrefe.

Halmer-Stein, R., Schmölz, A., Oberegelsbacher, D. and Gathmann, P. (1993). Music Therapy in Austria. In C. Dileo Maranto (ed.), *Music Therapy: International Perspectives (pp.63–88)*. Pipersville, PA: Jeffrey Books.

Hofbauer, S. (2015). Überblick: Kosten der Psychotherapie [Overview: Costs of psychotherapy]. Vienna: bestNET Information-Service. Retrieved from www.psyonline.at/contents/7437/ueberblick-kosten-der-psychotherapie on 15 May 2016.

Huffstutler, S.Y. and Varnell, G. (2006). The impostor phenomenon in new nurse practitioner graduates. *Topics in Advanced Practice Nursing eJournal*, 6, 2.

Koelsch, S. and Stegemann, T. (2012). The Brain and Positive Biological Effects in Healthy and Clinical Populations. In R. MacDonald, G. Kreutz and L. Mitchell (eds) *Music, Health and Well-Being (pp.436–456)*. Oxford: Oxford University Press.

Mithen, S. (2009). The music instinct: The evolutionary basis of musicality. *Neurosciences and Music III – Disorders and Plasticity. Annals of the New York Academy of Sciences*, 1169, 3–12.

Mössler, K. (2008a). *Update on music therapy in Austria*. Voices Resources. Retrieved from https://voices.no/community/?q=country-of-the-month/2008-update-music-therapy-austria on 15 May 2016.

Mössler, K. (2008b). *Wiener Beiträge zur Musiktherapie, Band 8: Wiener Schule der Musiktherapie. Von den Pionieren zur Dritten Generation (1957 bis heute)* [Viennese contributions to music therapy, Vol. 8: Viennese School of Music Therapy. From the pioneers to the third generation (1957 until nowadays)]. Vienna: Praesens.

Mössler, K. (2011). 'I am a psychotherapeutically oriented music therapist.' Theory construction and its influence on professional identity formation under the example of the Viennese School of Music Therapy. *Nordic Journal of Music Therapy*, 20, 155–184.

Musiktherapiegesetz [Music Therapists Act] (2016). Vienna: Legal Information System of the Republic of Austria. Retrieved from www.ris.bka.gv.at/GeltendeFassung.wxe?Abfrage=Bundesnormen&Gesetzesnummer=20005868 on 15 May 2016.

Oberhauser, S. (2016). Welcome statement on the Austrian Federal Ministry of Health and Women's Affairs' website. Retrieved from www.bmg.gv.at/home/EN/Home on 19 December 2016.

Priestley, M. (1975). *Music Therapy in Action*. New York: St Martin´s Press.

Ridder, H.M.O., Stige, B., Qvale, L.G. and Gold, C. (2013). Individual music therapy for agitation in dementia: An exploratory randomized controlled trial. *Aging and Mental Health*, 17, 667–678.

Ruud, E. (1980). *Hva er musikkterapi?* [What is Music Therapy?] Oslo: Gyldendal.

Statistics Austria (2015). Health Expenditure in Austria. Vienna: Statistics Austria. Retrieved from www.statistik.at/web_en/statistics/PeopleSociety/health/health_expenditure/index.html#index1 on 15 May 2016.

Stegemann, T., Fitzthum, E., Timmermann, T. and Schmidt, H.U. (2013). The status of state-approved music therapy training courses in the German-speaking countries including European developments. In Deutsche Musiktherapeutische Gesellschaft (ed.) *Music Therapy Annual, Vol. 9: Where Does Music Therapy Stand within the Health Care System? (pp.51–70)*. Wiesbaden: Reichert.

Stegemann, T., Mauch, C., Stein, V. and Romer, G. (2008). Zur Situation der Musiktherapie in der stationären Kinder- und Jugendpsychiatrie [The status of music therapy in inpatient child and adolescent psychiatry]. *Zeitschrift für Kinder- und Jugendpsychiatrie und Psychotherapie* 36, 255–263.

Stegemann, T., Schmidt, H.U., Fitzthum, E. and Timmermann, T. (2016). *Music Therapy Training Programmes in Europe: Theme and Variations.* Wiesbaden: Reichert.

Stige, B. and Aarø, L.E. (2012). *Invitation to Community Music Therapy.* New York: Routledge.

CHAPTER 5

Ethics, Marketing and Transparency

Stine Lindahl Jacobsen

Introduction

This chapter explores how therapists can strive for transparency, integrity and ethicality in public and private practices. Marketing private practice becomes ethical by being transparent about issues such as documentation, number and length of sessions, supervision and the setting of fees (Tudor 1998). This chapter also seeks to address some of the greatest challenges a therapist faces – ensuring integrity and quality while striving for the independence of our clients. My ideas and insights include an exploration of pertinent issues around the following topics, which are influenced by research studies and literature on private psychotherapy practice and public health care, and I will refer to these concurrently:

- transparency
- ethical marketing
- supervision
- fees
- client independence and length of therapy
- documentation.

Transparency

Transparency is at the heart of ethical practice. Transparency is understood as the availability of full information in cooperative and collective decision-making and as the lack of hidden agendas. It refers to a free and open exchange whereby the rules and reasons behind agreements are fair and clear to all participants. Pink (2012) proposes that any private practitioner or salesperson should be attuned to their 'customers' and clear with information, being honest, direct and transparent.

Much has happened since the idea of 'New Public Management' (NPM) was implemented in 1990s, in Denmark and the United Kingdom. NPM has been defined as 'a new (or renewed) stress on the importance of management and "production engineering" in public service delivery, which often linked to doctrines of economic rationalism' (Hood 1989; Pollitt 1993). In the UK and Denmark, it is questionable how effective NPM has been, as discussed by Hood and Dixon in their recent study (Hood & Dixon 2015). However, within health care, the line between private and state-provided therapy has become more invisible as the demands for transparency in these two different contexts has become more closely aligned, partly as a consequence of NPM ideas.

Aspiring to transparency can be very different in its implementation depending on the autonomy of the therapist. Private practitioners often have more freedom to set their own company values, create customised treatment plans, decide on supervision rates and revise budgets to fit cash flow requirements. Public sector practitioners rarely have the same level of freedom, and often operate in bureaucratic clinical services. There is a balance between the needs of the private practitioner, who needs to earn money to try to sustain the financial side of their practice, against the needs of the public sector practitioner who receives a steady monthly income, but has little or no responsibility or control over budgets, costs and profits. The impact of cutbacks and the demands of cost–benefit analyses from the state means public sector practitioners providing more transparent treatment plans. They must be able to document how much therapy is needed for clients and how much therapy is available depending on how many hours the therapist can provide. A public practitioner holds increasingly more responsibility in terms of ensuring transparency and documentation. If you cannot show the effect of your work or make the clinical argument for more or less therapy, you can potentially lose your job.

Private organisations working for profit and selling therapy need to rely on their reputation for quality as well as ensuring that their mission statement, policies and fee-setting procedures are transparent if they are to survive. If commissioners in the marketplace start to feel a particular company is too expensive or that they set their recommended length of or number of treatments unrealistically high or are in any other way unethical about service provision, this can adversely affect them, and may impact their survival. There are examples outside of the arts therapies which attest to the potential negative impact of market forces on the survival of companies. A clear framework is therefore required to ensure therapy organisations transparently determine:

- number of therapy sessions

- whether to stop or to continue treatment

- who is providing the therapy.

In some countries where the law allows it, word-of-mouth recommendations, written testimonials and descriptions of the therapy service can be used to enhance an organisation's reputation, and give an ethical overview of how a company runs its affairs.

Transparency also includes being open about the frequency of supervision and how often the therapists keep their training current within their field and individual expertise. In a public sector setting, the existence of the institution providing therapy services may not be threatened in the same way as a private company if the clinical set-up is not transparent and ethical. The state has 'approved' the public sector institution and clients may tend to trust their experts. Demand is rarely as high because public services are often free at the point of delivery, or at least less expensive. People tend to have higher expectations and demand more when they pay themselves (Clark & Sims 2014; Tudor 1998). This is not to question the quality of either private or public sector services, but simply to cast light on the demands and conditions in both settings. Ensuring ethical standards and therapist integrity is equally challenging regardless of the context of the working environment.

Ethical marketing

The American Marketing Association (2013) most recently defined marketing as 'the activity, set of institutions, and processes for creating, communicating, delivering, and exchanging offerings that have value for customers, clients, partners, and society at large'. Marketing is essential as it allows clients and commissioners to find the services they require. The onus is on the organisation or business to advertise their services in an ethical manner, ensuring the messages are not misleading. Private practitioners who market and sell therapy services to vulnerable people risk being seen as potentially unethical because of the hierarchical relationship between themselves and vulnerable clients. Exploiting vulnerable people using therapeutic skills to manipulate and lure them in for business reasons is deeply unethical and uncaring about the wellbeing of the potential client and their recovery (Clark & Sims 2014).

Public sector therapists are also required have initial consultative talks with potential clients, and do assessments prior to treatment. They therefore are open to the same risk of convincing potential clients that their particular form of therapy and approach is the absolute perfect match to the presenting condition. Within the private sector, such unethical and opaque practices cannot survive for long without serious damage to the reputation of the private company or private practitioner – or so we can hope.

In marketing therapy, suggesting treatment plans and modalities, inspiring commissioners and building partnerships, we must not only describe what we do and its potential effect or impact. As therapists we are very used to describing methods, interventions and techniques and we can fairly easily access literature and research publications supporting the positive effect of creative arts therapy. However, in truly striving for transparency in our marketing, we are called upon to include information about the context surrounding the possible therapy, helping to make the potential client truly understand what they are buying or receiving. This might seem painfully obvious, but in an internet search looking at websites of both private and public sector therapy providers, information about amount of supervision, how fees are set, access to continuing professional development (CPD) for therapists, and testimonials from former clients were often difficult to find.

Supervision

Clinical supervision is an essential part of ethical practice. The purpose of clinical supervision is to assist the practitioner to learn from their experience and progress in expertise, as well as to ensure good service to the client. In the UK, registered allied health professionals such as occupational therapists, physiotherapists, dieticians, speech and language therapists, and art, music and drama therapists are now expected to have regular clinical supervision of at least 1.5 hours a month (Bond 2013). From an international perspective, clinical supervision for practising therapists as a form of quality assurance is often a thorny issue. Depending on each country's regulatory framework and how well governance structures are organised, professional supervision or peer supervision can either be mandatory or an optional part of practice. It is the therapist's own responsibility, regardless of which setting they are in, to ensure their work is supervised. Supervision can also be understood as self-care. In certain countries clinical supervision may not be valued highly, as it is seen alongside less intense forms of self-care, including taking long walks, talking with peers and being 'good to yourself'. Some psychotherapists argue that clinical supervision is a growing challenge because of globalisation (Pettifor, Sinclair & Falender 2014). They recommend recognising supervision as a professional competence to ensure qualified and trained supervisors oversee clinical practice. Studies further stress the need to continue developing international clinical guidelines for supervision, and incorporating supervision in training programmes as a mandatory part of clinical work (Pettifor et al. 2014). A survey of the effect of music therapy supervision revealed a lack of quantitative research looking at the benefits of supervision on client outcomes. Such research would aid arguments in favour of professional supervision and possibly help both private and public sector practitioners to use supervision effectively, and highlight to clients supervision's valuable oversight role (Kennelly, Daveson & Baker 2015). Unfortunately, research suggests that psychotherapists do not always seek enough supervision and therefore do not have access to this form of quality assurance (Carney & Jefferson 2014). The findings of an American survey indicated that almost two-thirds of professional music therapists did not participate in supervision (Jackson 2008). In Australia, a 2012 survey found the two highest ranked reasons for not using supervision were working in a setting where supervision was 'not needed', and working with a population where supervision was 'not required' (Kennelly *et al.* 2012). Findings from a small survey of how private psychotherapy practitioners in the UK ensured suitable clinical support for their work showed that all of the 31 participants received and valued supervision. The private psychotherapists highlighted the need for external supervision because of the independent/lone-working nature of their practice, where isolation and exclusion were a risk (Savic-Jabrow 2010). For this research, it is clear that an ethical business, organisation or self-employed therapist should use regular clinical supervision to maintain quality assurance and client outcomes.

Due to the high variation in the use and understanding of clinical supervision amongst psychotherapists and creative arts therapists, across countries and settings, our individual stance towards supervision becomes even more important. Regardless of what supervision is understood to be, or what national/international ethical guidelines state, to ensure transparency when selling or inspiring people about access to therapy, current best practice indicates that we should inform our clients specifically about why and how often clinical supervision is used and how it plays an important role in ensuring quality.

Fees

Setting fees is no small matter when you run a private practice. Year-end turnover always needs to end up in profit, however small. Fees need to be stated and make sense to any customer, client, commissioner or relative. Setting fees is rarely something we need to worry about when working in public sector settings; nevertheless, as therapists use public tax revenues in the provision of therapy services, they still have a requirement to keep track of hours spent providing therapy, outcomes and customer satisfaction. This is useful when making the case for a pay raise or advocating how the service is worthwhile for clients.

Private practice is unique, however, in that it is only in this setting that therapists may experience a client or a commissioner asking for a discount or wanting to discuss the fee. Given the recent economic downturn, many practitioners are experiencing higher no-show rates, fewer new clients, and increased demand for negotiated fees (Colburn 2013). Setting fees is often a difficult area for private therapists, counsellors and creative arts therapists. Research shows that men are better at setting fees and dealing with queries than women and some practitioners argue that clients should only pay what they can afford (Myers 2008). If therapists set prices too low, they may create a barrier to providing high-quality services while making a sustainable profit, and risk burnout due to an inflated caseload to increase revenue. Low price typically begets low quality. High price typically begets high quality (Wright 2006).

However, according to Myers (2008), difficulties around setting fees could relate to ethical and therapist issues. Bringing the subject of money into the therapy room makes it personal rather than impersonal, political rather than neutral. Therapists have a tendency to want to be seen to give (to clients) without wanting to display or admit any kind of personal desire or need. Therapists might even wince at being accused of 'running a business' even though as private practitioners this is exactly what they do (Myers 2008). When a therapist asks for money, the client is put in a position where they have to recognise and acknowledge their need for therapy. Avoiding any challenging discussions with clients about discounts or an inability to pay may have more to do with the therapist's fear of increased engagement, the risk that the client will decide not to go ahead with therapy, and the risk of connecting with the 'real self' of the client. Even though it is difficult, we as therapists should talk with clarity to clients about money (Myers 2008). Surviving a discussion or conflict about money might even add to the vital dynamic processes in the client. Our willingness to have a transparent and open discussion about money and fees may also be a way of working towards greater client independence. By entering into such an intimate dialogue we may help clients in their struggle for more integrity and independence themselves. For both therapist and client, being independent means dealing with the fact that you are the source of your own income/resources which means having agency and a level of individual freedom which can offer many new possibilities and therapeutic change (Myers 2008).

Client independence and length of therapy

Ultimately the aim for any therapy should be that the need for treatment ends, allowing the client to become more independent and no longer in need of therapy. As therapists we need to aim for client independence, but this requires a high level of integrity. This is because when a client ends therapy, the therapist will also 'lose' income, which unless therapists ensure good new caseload flow ultimately means no income and no food on the table. When therapists set the number of sessions needed, they need to base their decision on more than a subjective evaluation, as they can be unconsciously biased towards keeping clients in therapy to ensure their own income.

A Danish PhD study examined how psychotherapy affects client independence and how often former clients seek help or contact the public health care system (Fenger 2012; Fenger *et al.* 2013). Over 700 clients with non-psychotic psychiatric problems such as depression, stress, anxiety and mild eating disorders were referred to a psychiatric unit in Denmark that participated in one part of the study. Collected through a large statistical database in Denmark, data from 15,200 randomly chosen people functioned as a matched control group. Out of the 761 participants who were offered psychotherapy, 545 accepted the treatment while 216 declined. Data was collected for the four years before treatment and every year in the four years following treatment (date of discharge from psychiatric hospital). The findings of the study show that clients who received psychotherapy had a significantly higher use of health care services than the control group. In another part of the study, findings showed that clients who received psychotherapy had a significantly higher amount of sick days and took earlier retirement than clients who did not receive psychotherapy during their stay at the psychiatric unit. The study questions how researchers measure effect as this evidence shows no equivalency between client independence from the health care system and fewer sick days. The finding also addresses the issue of using patient-reported outcomes to improve health care quality and not only medical database data (Hostetter & Klein 2012). The Fenger study further questions how psychotherapists work with client independence in our clinical methods and interventions. Do we like our client's dependency on us as therapists a little too much? So much so that we may actually want to keep them in therapy and make them seek more help even after discharge or end of treatment? Maybe therapists are subconsciously interested in clients being therapy-dependent and this is why we chose to be 'helpers' in the first place? It is hoped that this unhealthy mutual dependency relationship is not our intention, but we need to consciously take this into consideration when we plan and perform therapy. As creative arts therapists we often work with clients with severe problems such as autism, schizophrenia and multiple disabilities, and we know these clients will never be completely 'discharged'. However, with these client populations we still need to be aware of how we work towards client independence not only in the interventions themselves, but also in how we try to make ourselves indispensable and how we determine the amount of therapy needed. How do therapists decide this in an ethical manner? It might seem unfamiliar or challenging to think about treatment from the perspective of how much is enough rather than how much is needed for full recovery. However, if we rob the clients of their independence in the progress, by suggesting long-term therapy from the outset, we need to at least transparently consider what our real motivation may be.

Steering clear of unconscious dependency issues between client and therapist issues is a challenge in both private and public sector practice. Ensuring an ethical and unbiased evaluation of dose is an issue for all clinicians. In private practice the challenge is that you only answer to the client, their relatives or the commissioners, and with the therapist's role as an expert, it can seem fairly easy to argue for more therapy. However, with the increasing demand for transparency and increased access to information together with the impact of competition within the therapy marketplace, private clients and commissioners set high expectations and demands (Clark & Sims 2014; Tudor 1998). If they are not satisfied they will find alternative provision elsewhere and may not recommend you to others. If they are really displeased they might even contribute negatively to your reputation. A worst-case scenario could mean a therapist no longer has a private practice, as a poor reputation could directly affect the flow of new clients. In a public sector setting when therapists determine the treatment, they answer to the client, relatives and the employer. The same challenge of not exploiting your position as an expert does exist in this setting. Sometimes therapists need to follow fixed number of sessions regardless of what any subjective or objective documentation or assessment shows. This can make it very difficult to ensure integrity, transparency and flexibility based on each individual's actual presenting condition.

Massive cutbacks in public health care can put public sector psychotherapists and creative arts therapists under pressure as arguments are made that their services are 'nice to have' rather than 'need to have' when seen alongside medical, physiotherapy or psychiatric treatment. Ensuring a good flow of clients in public sector services might be out of an individual therapist's control. This actually makes an evaluation of client flow an even greater challenge. The risk of losing employment even when objective measures are used in documentation and treatment in a transparent and ethical manner is still present. Public sector therapists still worry about reputational issues but do not carry the sole responsibility for the service, elements of which may influence reputation. Regardless of the setting, taking care of client independence and setting the therapy requirements in an ethical and transparent manner requires a robust set of evaluation and documentation procedures and tools.

Documentation

Any public sector organisation or private practitioner has to uphold integrity by using some form of objective and reliable assessment or evaluation tool to set relevant goals and to monitor possible progress (Jacobsen, Wigram & Rasmussen 2014). When marketing therapy services, explaining how the therapist or the organisation determines what type and how much therapy may be required is critical. Organisations and therapists need to be seen to be treating clients with respect and providing the best service possible for clinical and ethical reasons. Clients need to understand what they are buying. Therapists want clients to feel able to come back for additional therapy support and add positively to reputational awareness of the service. Both these help to keep therapy businesses running, and enable other clients to benefit from good-quality therapy in the future (Pink 2012).

Validated assessment tools can offer objective insights into the type and severity of problems for both clients and clinicians. As a private practitioner, having objective information next to a valuable subjective or individualised assessment procedure can aid decision-making processes (Jacobsen *et al.* 2014). If the two set of data disagree, digging deeper, readjusting, inviting client or relatives into the discussion and focusing your approach to meet the clinical problem at hand may enhance reputation and improve clinical effectiveness. If the two sets of information agree, therapists can feel confident about their approach and more willing to share information with the client.

When thinking about ending therapy or extending it, how should a psychotherapist or creative arts therapist use integrity and ethical transparency to argue for continuation or cessation of therapy? If they implement tools to document change or if they provide thorough service evaluations, they will have stronger arguments for either recommendation depending on the outcome (Mellor-Clark et al. 2014). Clients and commissioners will be able to see if therapy is targeting the right areas or not, and if the therapy has a positive effect or not, and it will be based on more than a subjective professional and possibly biased evaluation. Objective documentation serves as strong arguments for either continuing or ending therapy, both for private practitioners and public sector practitioners. Explaining to clients how evaluation and a determination of therapeutic input is arrived at supports transparency. Some clients might not be able to engage in such explanations but nevertheless, is it necessary to have access to such information, to ensure quality in your clinical approach (Mellor-Clark *et al.* 2014). Using validated tools can be quite complex and often requires additional training to become certified to use them in clinical practice. Training is expensive but it should be seen as a matter of investment that adds to the quality of the therapeutic service (Jacobsen *et al.* 2014).

Using research publications to argue for the positive effect of creative arts therapy or psychotherapy for different client groups is also relevant in maintaining transparent practice. Often research provides useful information about the number of sessions needed to ensure positive effect. However, every setting and approach is different and nobody can guarantee a positive therapeutic effect. Research results must be used with integrity and transparency. There is a great difference between promising positive effects and explaining the probability of positive effects (Teachman *et al.* 2012). Recommendations from other clients and commissioners might serve as the best way to openly state the quality of an approach or a therapist's particular work (Pink 2012).

Within public sector services, documenting therapists' own clinical practice and therapeutic approach is worthwhile even though the immediate concern is not sustaining budgets and reputation management. Public institutions also need to know whether the therapy is targeting planned aims, and whether clients are getting better, or at least not getting worse. This is not to say we shouldn't end therapy if there is no positive change in symptoms or continue it if there is positive change. Of course we use our professional expertise and consider any relevant contextual information about the client regardless of the public or private nature of each setting. But by using external and/or objective information or data to help support therapeutic decisions, we increase integrity both within the field of creative arts therapy and as individual therapists.

As stated earlier, private psychotherapy practitioners may be better able to target new client flow more effectively than public sector practitioners. In private practice marketing, there may be more freedom to focus on what is believed to be a relevant challenge for the organisation, and not what public services want you to take on as a therapist regardless of your professional competences. Targeting clients to fit your clinical skills is one way of ensuring integrity and quality, but diversifying therapy with a team of private therapists also has benefits, such as increasing revenue, improving business resilience, flexible work schedules, more clients, enhanced skills and more connections (Colburn 2013). Adapting to clinical and environmental changes and making customised treatment plans seems more accessible for private practitioners than public sector practitioners. Psychotherapists working with a public sector service do not carry the heavy burden of financial responsibility, although they may collect helpful and necessary data relevant to financial decisions and choices required by the increasing demand for documentation within these sectors (Hood & Dixon 2015). Private practitioners have financial responsibility but they also have the freedom to ensure quality, integrity and ethical transparency by customising treatment plans and targeting client flow.

Conclusion

By maintaining integrity and ethics in marketing and advertising therapy services, or arguing for an extension to therapy provision, the contextual set-up around the therapy must be transparent. This helps clients and/or commissioners clearly understand what they are buying. Both in private and public sector practice this includes information about the specific competences of the therapists, frequency of supervision, setting the number of sessions and fees, documentation procedures, the frequency of CPD, and preferably recommendations from former clients and users. All practitioners need to strive for a level of client independence that seems appropriate for the individual client and must not be biased towards wanting to maintain their job or unconsciously holding on to an interdependent client–therapist relationship.

Discussions about fee-setting with clients are often necessary but can challenge the therapist's sense of identity. However, keeping an authentic stance and an open dialogue with clients can actually aid the therapeutic process and further strengthen client independence. Using validated assessment tools and relying on effect research can further add to a transparent practice where most clinical decisions are backed up by objective information or probability of prognosis.

Aiming for transparency is equally challenging for private and public sector practitioners. It is hard work and no one can claim to be more or less ethical based solely on their setting. It entirely depends on choices made by each therapist and their own level of integrity. However, one might speculate on who has more opportunity to ensure transparency and integrity – public sector or private practitioners? The level of freedom in private practice seems to increase possibilities to establish and prioritise quality assurance through regular supervision, CPD, targeted client flow, usage of validated evaluation tools, high-standard documentation procedures, and so on. Of course, this freedom is only accessible if the private practitioner manages to develop enough profit in their annual budget to afford to make these investments. The private practitioner might equally choose to spend any profit on a nice Ferrari instead of investing in business by establishing quality assurance and a transparent practice.

The reputation of such a private practitioner might suffer a great deal if the service lacks quality and transparency and we can only hope that such enterprises do not exist for very long. Compared with public sector practitioners, there is almost no choice for the individual practitioner not to prioritise quality assurance. As a public sector psychotherapist or arts therapist you might be employed at an institution where integrity, transparency and ethics are commonplace. However, in the same institution, there may be much uncertainty about your employment, with you having little control over work tasks and client flow. Ideally, a setting where the therapist can be authentic in their approach and show independence in their relationships with clients, thereby being inspired by and taking responsibility in creating solid clinical practice, seems preferable. Building a business to call your own and keeping it alive might be one way to ensure such a stance, but actively engaging in decisions, making demands and setting limits in public institutions should always be as transparent and successful in striving for true client independence and transparent practice.

Go and do it!

Exercise 1: Qualities of a therapist/service

What would you demand to know about the therapist and the company/public service before you or a family member could feel safe about entering therapy? Describe this to a fellow therapist/student to try to see the perspective of the clients and their families when you want a transparent provider of therapy.

Exercise 2: Fee discussions

Role play fee discussions with clients and relatives to find your outer limits and to feel confident in having these discussions. The client and relatives should have different levels of maturity and different clinical issues in order for you to enhance your skills and gain greater insights into your individual therapist identity.

Exercise 3: Documentation

Role play describing how you document your clinical work in a transparent and clear manner to commissioners, clients and relatives.

References

American Marketing Association (2013). About AMA. Retrieved from www.ama.org/AboutAMA/Pages/Definition-of-Marketing.aspx on 10 January 2017.

Bond, T. (2013). *Ethical Framework for Good Practice in Counselling and Psychotherapy*. Leicestershire: British Association for Counselling and Psychotherapy.

Carney, J.M. and Jefferson, J.F. (2014). Consultation for mental health counsellors: Opportunities and guidelines for private practice. *Journal of Mental Health Counselling*, 36, 4, 302–314.

Clark, P. and Sims, P.L. (2014). The practice of fee setting and collection: Implications for clinical training programs. *American Journal of Family Therapy*, 42, 5, 386–397.

Colburn, A.A.N. (2013). Endless possibilities: Diversifying service options in private practice. *Journal of Mental Health Counselling*, 35, 3, 198–210.

Fenger, M.M. (2012). *Psychotherapy: Attendance and effects on utilisation of health care services and occupational functioning*. PhD thesis, Copenhagen University, Copenhagen.

Fenger, M.M., Poulsen, S., Mortensen, E.L. and Lau, M. (2013). A register-based study of occupational functioning in non-psychotic patients before and after psychotherapy. *Open Psychiatry Journal*, 7, 1–8.

Hood, C. (1989). Public administration and public policy: Intellectual challenges for the 1990s. *Australian Journal of Public Administration*, 48, 346–358.

Hood, C. and Dixon, R. (2015). *A Government that Worked Better and Cost Less? Evaluating Three Decades of Reform and Change in UK Central Government*. New York: Oxford University Press.

Hostetter, M. and Klein, S. (2012). Using patient-reported outcomes to improve health care quality. *Quality Matters Archive*. Retrieved from www.commonwealthfund.org/publications/newsletters/quality-matters/2011/december-january-2012/in-focus on 27 May 2016.

Jackson, N. (2008). Professional music therapy supervision: A survey. *Journal of Music Therapy*, 45, 2, 192–216.

Jacobsen, S.L., Wigram, T. and Rasmussen, A.M. (2014) Assessment – klinisk vurdering i musikterapi [Assessment – clinical evaluation in music therapy]. In Bonde (ed.) *Musikterapi – teori – uddannelse – forskning – praksis* [music therapy – theory – education – research – practice] (pp.310–332). Copenhagen: Hans Reitzels Forlag.

Kennelly, J.D., Baker, F.A., Morgan, K.A. and Daveson, B.A. (2012). Supervision for music therapists: An Australian cross-sectional survey regarding views and practices. *Australian Journal of Music Therapy*, 23, 41–56.

Kennelly, J.D., Daveson, B.A. and Baker, F.A. (2015). Effects of professional music therapy supervision on clinical outcomes and therapist competency: A systematic review involving narrative synthesis. *Nordic Journal of Music Therapy*. doi: 10.1080/08098131.2015.1010563.

Mellor-Clark, J., Cross, S., Macdonald, J. and Skjulsvik, T. (2014) Leading horses to water: Lessons from a decade of helping psychological therapy services use routine outcome measurement to improve practice. *Administration and Policy in Mental Health and Mental Health Service* 43, 3, 279–285.

Myers, K. (2008). Show me the money: (The 'problem' of) the therapist's desire, subjectivity and relationship to the fee. *Contemporary Psychoanalysis*, 44, 118–140.

Pettifor, J., Sinclair, C. and Falender, C.A. (2014). Ethical supervision: Harmonizing rules and ideals in a globalizing world. *Training and Education in Professional Psychology* 8, 4, 201–210. Retrieved from http://dx.doi.org/10.1037/tep0000046 on 28 November 2016.

Pink, D.H. (2012). *To Sell is Human. The Surprising Truth about Moving Others*. New York: Riverhead Books.

Pollitt, C. (1993). *Managerialism and the Public Services* (2nd edition). Oxford: Blackwell.

Savic-Jabrow, P.C. (2010). Where do counsellors in private practice receive their support? A pilot study. *Counselling and Psychotherapy Research*, 10, 3, 229–232.

Teachman, B.A., Drabick, D.A.G., Hershenberg, R., Vivian, D., Wolfe, B.E. and Goldfried, M. (2012). Bridging the gap between clinical research and clinical practice: Introduction to the special section. *Psychotherapy, 49,* 2, 97–100.

Tudor, K. (1998). Value for money?: The issues of fees in counselling and psychotherapy. *British Journal of Guidance and Counselling,* 26, 4, 477–493.

Wright, M.R. (2006). Setting appropriate fees. *Optometry and Vision Development,* 37, 1, 19–20.

CHAPTER 6

Educating Students
Getting Ready for the Job Market
Petra Kern

Introduction

During the final year of undergraduate studies in the USA, students typically ask questions about their professional employment prospects and best fit in the workforce. Based on their competencies, interests, values, personal characteristics, and financial capacities, three career paths may present themselves as an option: graduate studies and academia, employment by an agency, institute, or organization, or self-employment and private practice. When exploring entrepreneurship, students often lack knowledge and experience on how to start and succeed in private practice and may have questions, as outlined in Figure 6.1.

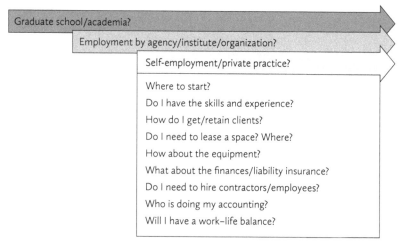

Figure 6.1 Career options and questions for healthcare undergraduate students

While many healthcare undergraduate programs prepare students to be effective evidence-based practitioners, little time may actually be devoted to the business aspect of therapy and how to make a living practicing one's chosen profession. After graduation and passing the board-certification exam, numerous young professionals enter the workforce with a limited understanding that business success relies on a different set of competencies and tools than does therapy. Hence, what seems to be missing in the undergraduate curriculum is instruction on how to succeed as a healthcare entrepreneur – knowledge that is vital to compete in today's business world (Behnke 1996; Guy 2005; Lacy & Hadsell 2003; Tonkinson 2014; Wilhelm 2004).

Starting with the importance of business skills for healthcare providers, this chapter focuses on a five-week project teaching entrepreneurship to students who are about to join the workforce. Topics include understanding basic concepts in building a business, collaborating with potential business partners in setting up a private practice, evaluating current developments and trends, meeting with experts, applying services and resources that are available from university-based career development centers, and peer coaching. Examples of music therapy business modules, student activities, and reflective statements illustrate the content of this chapter.

Teaching for success

The success of higher education degree programs should not only be based on academic achievements, but also on immediate employment, competitive salaries, job satisfaction, and occupation retention of alumni. Thus, it is essential for educators to be informed about outcomes of current employment trend analysis, organizational workforce data, and job opportunities in the field. Competing with other professionals, educators must prepare students for the job market by making a priority of embedding current developments and trends in a curriculum that prepares them for today and tomorrow (Global Business School Network 2013; Selingo 2013; Udacity 2016).

For example, an employment trend analysis in music therapy conducted by Silverman and Furman (2014) revealed that between 1998 and 2009, 500 more music therapy positions (mainly in schools; kindergarten to 12th grade), nursing homes, and self-employment/private practice) have been created in the USA. Next to school settings, self-employment and private practice ranked as the second highest work setting for music therapists – a trend that can also be observed in the growing number of music therapy business websites, blogs, and Facebook fan pages. The researchers conclude, 'From the large numbers of music therapists working in self-employment/private practice, it would seem appropriate for university programs to prepare students to institute and administer new businesses' (p.107).

Given that many graduates will enter the workforce as healthcare entrepreneurs, teaching basic business skills should be a key component in every curriculum. Professional organizations such as the American Music Therapy Association (AMTA 2013, 2014, 2015) or the Certification Board of Music Therapists (2016) should outline in their documents their professional competencies, board certification domains, scope of practice, and code of ethics, more detailed proficiencies and ways to conduct business. Furthermore, essential business skills should be included in the course of study (e.g. basic planning, designing, financing, bookkeeping/accounting, marketing/advertising, documenting, and balancing work and life). In summary, a successful career in private practice requires more than being a competent therapist. As therapy is a profession, any new healthcare entrepreneur—whether as solo business owner or business partner—must understand business models and operations in order to thrive.

Designing the course

The following description of the business segment is based on an undergraduate course (i.e. MUTH 432-01: Principles and Practices of Music Therapy II) piloted over three years in the music therapy program at the University of Louisville. This competence-based course segment was delivered in hybrid format (i.e. on campus and online), including in-class discussions, real-life examples, expert advice, peer coaching, experimental elements, and engaging weekly assignments. While examples represent information and works from the music therapy field, content and concepts can be adjusted to undergraduate and graduate studies in related healthcare disciplines.

Learning outcomes

As with planning any course, identifying clear learning outcomes that are closely linked with professional competencies requirements is crucial for successful teaching (Palloff & Pratt 2013). Specific to the business segment, students in this music therapy undergraduate course were expected to achieve the following learning outcomes:

- understand the basic concepts of building your own business

- collaborate with potential business partners in setting up a music therapy business

- evaluate the music therapy industry and the current climate and trends

- network and learn from experts in the field

- identify your transferrable skills and make use of available resources

- use technology and media for marketing, and

- reflect on your qualities and confidence as a potential entrepreneur.

Weekly course objectives, readings and resources, instructions, and assignments posted on the course management system (i.e. Blackboard) reflected the learning outcomes set for this business segment of the course. Students were expected to engage with the course content through individual work and teamwork. The instructor monitored the students' learning processes and supported them in achieving the learning outcomes through onsite teaching, online meetings, and ongoing feedback.

Readings and resources

At the time, no textbook about 'the business of therapy' was available. However, there are several 'how to' books, articles, reports, and audio podcasts published by music therapists and other healthcare providers. For this course segment, music therapy students were required to use the workbook *The Therapy Business Blueprint* by Kimberly Sena Moor (2008). Students were also expected to listen to audio podcasts and review recommended resources that supported their individual and team assignments. Examples are displayed in Table 6.1.

Table 6.1 Audio podcasts and recommended resources

Audio podcasts	AMTA.Pro. (producer) (2012, August). *Barbara Reuer: Mover and Shaker*. http://amtapro.musictherapy.org/?p=963#more-963.
	AMTA.Pro. (producer) (2011, August). *Meredith Pizzi: Making it Work – MT-BC and Small Business Owner*. http://amtapro.musictherapy.org/?p=739.
	Lindstrom, J. (producer) (2012, April 17). *Tim Ringgold: Start-out-successful*. www.blogtalkradio.com/mtshow/2012/01/27/tim-ringgold-start-out-successful.
	Music Therapy Round Table. Business-related episodes. http://musictherapyroundtable.com.
	Sena Moore, K. (author) (2016, October 1). *Creating Capacity: What Music Therapists Need to Know about Starting a Private Practice*. www.imagine.musictherapy.biz/?page_id=5.
Recommended resources	American Music Therapy Association (2015). *2015 AMTA Member Survey and Workforce Analysis: A Descriptive Statistical Profile of the AMTA Membership*. Silver Spring, MD: AMTA.
	Apple (2016). *iMovie: Turn your videos into movie magic*. www.apple.com/ilife/imovie.
	Career Development Center (2016). *Music Careers in Dollars and Cents*. Boston, MA: Berklee College of Music.
	Fulton, K. (producer) (2011, September 15). *Music Therapists Talk about Self-Care: A Video Interview* [video podcast]. www.imagine.musictherapy.biz/?p=901#more-901.
	Ggrodzki, L. (2015). *Building Your Ideal Private Practice: A Guide for Therapists and Other Healing Professionals* (2nd edition). New York: W.W. Norton & Company Ltd.
	Knoll, C. and Henry, D. (2014). *You're the Boss! Self-employment Strategies for Music Therapists*. Stephenville, TX: MusicWorksPublication.com.
	Pizzi, M. and Guy, J. (eds.) (2015). *Leading the Way—Music Therapy Business of the Future: A Workbook*. Silver Spring, MD: AMTA.
	Rambach, R. (2011). Building your own business in early childhood music therapy. *imagine*, 2, 1, 90.
	Silverman, M.J., Furman, A.G., Schwartzberg, E.T., Leonard, J., Stephens, E. and McKee, R. (2013). Music therapy salaries from 1998–2012: A comparative and descriptive study. *Music Therapy Perspectives*, 31, 4, 181–188.
	Simpson, J. and Burns, D.S. (2004). *Music Therapy Reimbursement: Best Practices and Procedures*. Silver Spring, MD: AMTA.
	US Small Business Administration (n.d.) Build Your Business Plan. www.sba.gov/tools/business-plan/1.

Business segment

The business segment began with an onsite 'Weekend Intensive Course.' Students read the e-book by Sena Moore (2008) and prepared the following three questions for an initial in-class discussion: (1) What are pros and cons of self-employment, especially for newcomers in the field? (2) Which music therapy private businesses capture your attention and why?, and (3) How would you get started with building your own business? After a lively topic 'kick-off,' students engaged with the content of the workbook by exploring the seven-step procedure, expanded with in-class activities and personalized examples described as follows.

Step 1: What do you want?

This step explores the fundamental question about the potential business owner's ultimate purpose in life and primary life goal, the Definite Major Purpose (DMP). The reasons are twofold: (1) to evaluate life-fulfilling personal and professional success, and (2) to have clarity for decision-making and goal achievement. Writing down one's own DMP and factors that bring satisfaction and fulfillment is suggested as the most important step in planning one's own business and determining if it is the right career path to pursue.

Activities and examples: In small teams, students discussed their personal life-fulfilling factors, explored the DMP statements of therapists who are business owners, and jotted down a first draft of their DMP statement. A DMP example shared by the instructor, who is the owner of the California-based company Music Therapy Consulting, was 'to enhance lives through music by providing music therapy consulting, coaching, and teaching to communities, parents, and students.'

Step 2: Build your team

This step stresses that specific expertise needed to build a private practice should be handed over to skillful professionals (e.g. attorney – helping with the business structure and other legal aspects; bookkeeper – maintenance of financial records; accountant – creating reports; graphic designer – creating an image and brand for the business; administrative assistant – taking care of mundane tasks). Hiring the services allows the new business owner to devote more time for providing services and creating products. That said, looking for more cost-effective alternatives might be necessary, especially when getting started.

Activities and examples: While discussing the importance of hiring professionals for specific business-related tasks, students explored alternative business tools outlined under resources by Sena Moore (2008), Rambach (2011), Pizzi and Guy (2015), and others. Examples included online business tools (e.g. Wordpress, PayPal, QuickBooks Online) and productivity apps (e.g. ical, square, kashoo).

Step 3: Define your identity

This step addresses the different types of names for businesses (e.g. personal name, regional association, sensory association, therapeutic association, scientific association, or a combination) and legal structure (e.g. sole proprietorship, partnerships, S- or C-corporation, limited liability company, and non-profit). While the business name defines the image and brand that draws clients, the legal business type defines the structure and liability of the business. There are various pros and cons for choosing one type of business name or legal structure over others—all need to be considered on an individual basis.

Activities and examples: Two student groups competed in searching the web for the best existing business name under each category. Examples shared were Bolton Music Therapy (personal name), Coast Music Therapy (regional association), Raising Harmony (sensory association), UofL Music Therapy Center (therapeutic association), Center for Biomedical Research in Music (scientific association), and Neurosong (a combination).

Step 4: Figure out financials

This step tackles ways to get paid for therapeutic services (e.g. private pay, grants, insurance/waiver reimbursement/Medicaid/Medicare). Basic accounting and bookkeeping terms (e.g. cash/accrual account, invoices, assets, liabilities, equity/capital/net worth, accounts receivable, accounts payable, chart of accounts, income and expense reports, balance sheets, and payroll) are important to learn for new business owners. Getting organized by opening a small business checking account, finding the right bookkeeper/accountant or software, creating a filing system, and setting up a regular schedule to maintain administrative tasks are key in streamlining the operation of the business.

Activities and examples: Using the recommended resources, students were to find facts to answer the following three questions: (1) What is the average annual income of a music therapist in your state? (2) What is the going rate for assessment, individual sessions, and group sessions for music therapy services in your state?, and (3) What are your major questions related to reimbursement of music therapy services in your state? As an example, students cited results from Silverman *et al.* (2013) (e.g. average income: USD $44,415.25; assessment rate: $93.23; individual session rate: $55.13; and group session rate: $53.71), and prepared sample questions for the reimbursement representative of the American Music Therapy Association whom they contacted later in the course.

Step 5: Prepare your paperwork

This step describes the importance of contracts (i.e. agreement between two or more parties), documentation (e.g. client progress), and invoices (e.g. payment of service) as communication tools. A basic contract should include policies and procedures, and rights and responsibilities (e.g. description of services, schedule, payment, absence and cancellations, term of agreement, rights and responsibilities, and acknowledgement and consent form). Furthermore, professional responsibilities of a therapist and business owner include documentation of the therapeutic process (e.g. referral, assessment, intervention plan, progress notes, evaluation/termination reports) and creating an invoice (e.g. a bill that includes the business's/client's name and contact information, the date, a description of the service provided—with date, type, and cost for each service, the total amount due, and the methods of payment by a set date).

Activities and examples: After reviewing various contract and documentation samples, students created an invoice for imaginary music therapy services using a template from Microsoft Project Gallery/Pages Template Chooser.

Step 6: Be a marketing maven

This step addresses effective marketing strategies (e.g. go where your target customers are, be helpful, listen, expand your network, always be nice, and be patient) and common marketing tools (e.g. business cards, websites, postcards/brochures, e-newsletter, media releases, social media, and word of mouth). Creating value for clients and building strong client relationships are key to a successful business. Choosing marketing tools for specific purposes that resonate with the target client group will be most effective.

Activities and examples: Students discussed, from a client perspective, which music therapy business owners' marketing strategies and tools were most appealing. Additionally, they created their first business card by using a free template from Vistaprint (www.vistaprint.com). The instructor shared examples of well-designed business cards. The students later used their new business cards for networking purposes at the regional and national music therapy conference.

Step 7: Final touches

This step discusses the legal environment (e.g. business license or permit, professional liability insurance, trademarks, copyright, domain names), the location (e.g. music therapy room or natural environment), equipment and materials (e.g. music instruments, computer and software, office supplies, and filing systems), personnel (e.g. employees, interns, and volunteers), and professional development (e.g. books/articles, conferences, online courses, and supervision). Each of the listed items need to be in order before the doors for business can open. Planning ahead will subsidize a healthy work–life balance.

Activities and examples: Students looked into the recommended liability insurance of the professional organization, viewed examples of well-equipped music therapy rooms, considered the advantages of becoming an approved internship provider, and evaluated professional development options. As an example for self-care practices, students viewed the video podcast *Music Therapists Talk about Self-Care: A Video Interview* (Fulton 2011).

At the end of the Weekend Intensive Course students were divided into small teams. First, student teams worked on a plan outlining action items, responsibilities, and deadlines for each task. In the following four weeks, student teams met for three course hours per week and worked together in accomplishing the course objectives outlined for each module. Weekly assignments were designed to revisit readings and resources and independently engage students with the course content. Resources outlined in Figure 6.2 provided support in mastering the expected tasks. The instructor made sure that all team members contributed equally and monitored the quality and timeliness of the deliverables. While weekly stand-up reports (i.e. video-based three-minute summaries of each student's contribution) posted on the course site's blog assisted in making all students accountable for their work, student teams and the instructor both called for additional online meetings as needed.

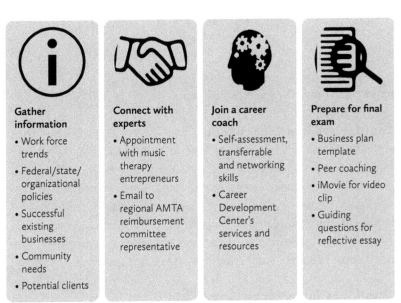

Gather information	Connect with experts	Join a career coach	Prepare for final exam
• Work force trends • Federal/state/organizational policies • Successful existing businesses • Community needs • Potential clients	• Appointment with music therapy entrepreneurs • Email to regional AMTA reimbursement committee representative	• Self-assessment, transferrable and networking skills • Career Development Center's services and resources	• Business plan template • Peer coaching • iMovie for video clip • Guiding questions for reflective essay

Figure 6.2 Resources for competence-based learning modules

Module 1: Gather information

Exploring questions outlined in Figure 6.3, students evaluated the healthcare sector and looked into current developments and trends by searching for workforce trend analyses, reviewing federal, state, and organizational policies, studying services and products from exciting music therapy businesses, and exploring local community needs. Then they identified potential clients (e.g. specific populations, agencies, institutions, and organizations) while brainstorming about the services and products they could provide based on their competencies, experiences, and professional scope of practice. Generally, students identified their unique niche for their prospective business.

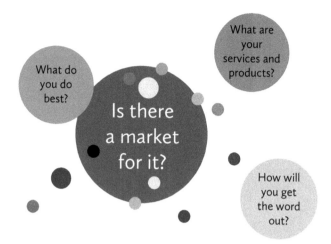

Figure 6.3 Brainstorming questions in preparation for writing a business plan

Revisiting course-related readings and resources, students then applied information relevant to their unique businesses. As a team, they discussed (1) their combined DMP, (2) services they need to hire, (3) the business name and structure they wanted to use, (4) available funding options in their state, (5) suitable contracts and documentation templates to use, (6) effective marketing strategies, and (7) legal documents, location, equipment, personnel, and mentoring needed to launch their first music therapy private practices.

Module 2: Connect with experts

Each student team had the opportunity to meet a music therapy entrepreneur who has a thriving business in the USA. Students prepared questions that arose during their information-gathering phase and met the assigned experts online or at the conferences of AMTA. While students expressed excitement to have expert exposure, the music therapy entrepreneurs also responded very positively. When asked about their motivation to share their business knowledge and expertise with students, which questions from students they found most interesting, and what they hope for the students when entering the business world, the music therapy entrepreneurs replied as follows:

> As a new graduate starting a private practice, the mentorship I received from experienced music therapy entrepreneurs was extremely valuable, which is why I try to provide the same to students and

young professionals now. I admired that students asked about my future plans and goals for my business and were interested in the 'big picture' perspective. I hope that the students are able to keep that 'big picture' mentality as they venture into the business world, and [will] always be working towards the next step. (Rachel Rambach, MM, MT-BC, owner of Music Therapy Connections, LLC)

When I was a student, I remember thinking I would never go into business for myself, because the idea terrified me. Now, as a music therapy entrepreneur, I love speaking to students to encourage them that private practice is a realistic option. I was glad that the students asked many questions about insurance reimbursement, as that is a huge avenue to increasing access to music therapy services for many clients. For the students that do go into private practice, I hope that they will take advantage of ongoing business training opportunities to hone their skills and sustain successful businesses. (Dana Bolton, MEd, MMT, MT-BC, owner of Bolton Music Therapy)

I enjoy the excitement that students have for the growing field of music therapy and love sharing ways to ethically grow our businesses. The students' social media marketing questions were interesting to me as it is important to consider ramifications of interacting through online means. My hope is that students will first seek employment to gain experience and avoid costly mistakes of being a newly self-employed provider in the field. (Jennifer Puckett, LPMT, MT-BC, owner of Therabeat, Inc.)

Additionally, student teams were invited to send an email to a representative of the AMTA reimbursement committee to ask specific questions about funding and reimbursement options for their prospective services. The experts' real-life examples and advice were invaluable for students. Not only did they help them in preparing their business ideas, they also encouraged them to explore private practice as possible career paths.

Module 3: Join the career coach

The university's Career Development Center encourages the faculty to partner and embed their services into the coursework. To take advantage of this opportunity, a career coach was invited to address the following topics during a coaching session: developing solid self-knowledge related to career choices and work performance; identifying and using strong transferrable skills; and building effective networking skills. Additionally, students were introduced to, and encouraged to use, the university's career services and resources. Finally, all students posted on the course site's blog a text-based summary and comment to a peer about what they had learned from the career coach and how they would apply the information and their identified talents for building their own businesses.

Module 4: Prepare for final exam

For the final exam, student teams first applied their newly gained knowledge and innovative ideas by preparing a business plan. Using the template of the US Small Business Administration (n.d.), students addressed the following business plan components: Title Page, Table of Contents, Executive Summary, Business Description and Vision, Definition of the Market, Description of Products and Services, Organization and Management, Marketing and Sales Strategy, Financial Management, and Appendices. Each section presented a short description of major points to be addressed, supporting students in focusing on specific goals and objectives.

Second, each student team pitched their business proposals in 'Shark Tank' style to a panel of business school students. The business school students asked team members in-depth questions, appraised each proposal, and identified the best pitch. Subsequently, the business school students provided peer coaching to strengthen each team's music therapy business proposal. An impression of the successful collaboration between the School of Music and College of Business at the University of Louisville, including the students' takeaways, can be viewed at Kern (2016).

Third, student teams created a three-minute video clip telling a convincing story about their music therapy business, highlighting the 'who, what, when, where, how, and why.' Students used a project theme from iMovie as a video creation and editing tool, and included a jingle or musical piece, images, and text underlining the message they wanted to convey to potential clients in the community. Students were encouraged to identify and make use of team members' talents, while contributing equally to the video project. An example of students' work can be accessed at Kern (2014b).

Fourth, students read the book by Grodzki (2015) and wrote a short reflective essay. The essay spoke to the following guiding questions: (1) Which strategies and ideas resonated most with you? (2) What surprising facts did you find in the text? (3) Which qualities and confidence level do you bring to building your own business? (4) In conclusion, is building your own business something you wish to pursue?

Additionally, students also reflected their individual learning outcomes, the course content, and delivery of the business segment during an online meeting with the instructor.

Assessment and evaluation

Addressing various learning styles, students were given the opportunity through discussions, writings, presentations, technology, and media assignments to demonstrate the set learning outcomes for the business course segment. Weekly assignments and deliverables led to the final exam submissions of a business plan, video clip, and reflective essay. The evaluation rubrics reflected attendance and active participation, the completeness and quality of work, creativity and innovation as well as time and size limits for media submissions. Assignment #4 (see the Appendix to this chapter for more details) outlines an example of learning outcomes, due dates, a step-by-step description, and evaluation rubrics, which can be adjusted to impending business course segments.

Keeping students accountable for their work and learning progress as well as equally contributing to teamwork needs to be monitored and reinforced. For this course segment, the following three components have proven to be successful: allocated teaming locations (onsite and online) and times; posting weekly stand-up reports; and peer ratings. Nevertheless, as technology develops, stronger tools in measuring accountability and student participation may become available in the near future.

Reflecting students' development

The achievement of the learning outcomes was evident by the students' works and reflective comments. Students mastered basic business skills and felt empowered by having a better understanding of the music therapy job market. For some students, self-employment and private practice became a realistic career option; others determined this might not be the best choice for them. The following comments provide a synopsis of students' impressions of the five-week business course segment.

> This course has helped me solidify my dream of opening a music therapy private practice one day and has made it seem more realistic and within reach. (Bailey Carter, MTS University of Louisville)

> The thought of opening my own private practice has always seemed very intimidating to me. However, after taking this course I now have the basic tools necessary to not only understand the inner workings of a private practice, but also to have the option to open one myself in a few years. (Emily Lobeck, MTS University of Louisville)

> This course gave me insight into the business side of music therapy that I would not have otherwise had. Regardless of any plans to go into business for myself, I feel better equipped to speak with both music therapists and business owners, which will be an important tool for networking. (Kyle McCammon, MTS University of Louisville)

> This course taught me that managing a music therapy business is a multidimensional process. It requires market research, clinical expertise, continuous adaptation and development of business goals, and creativity to successfully market and sell the service. Learning all of this has made me excited to take on the challenge of pursuing a business in music therapy after graduation. (Holly Hankin, MTS University of Louisville)

> This course segment gave me a greater understanding of what it means to be an entrepreneur. The skills that I have gained are not only needed to open a private practice, but also to start a music therapy program anywhere. (Garrett Weeks, MTS)

> After creating and pitching a business proposal in 'Shark Tank' style and receiving feedback from business students, the idea of opening a music therapy business seems less daunting and more feasible than I had initially thought! Even if I never start a business, the skills and knowledge gained through this course will serve me well throughout my career. (Madison Whelan, MTS University of Louisville)

What I have learned in this course allows me to better understand what is happening in the field of music therapy. It gives me an advantage over students who are not taught business skills and makes me more confident to become a successful music therapist. (Kelsey Norris, MTS University of Louisville)

In a video interview with three previous course participants (Kern 2014a), students responded to the following questions: (1) What was your 'aha' moment when learning about music therapy business skills?; (2) How did the team project contribute to your learning?; and (3) In which way did the topic influence your current and future thinking about your career? Following up with the alumni featured in this video revealed that one student applied for a Master's in Business Administration program to advance her knowledge in running a successful business. Another alumnus currently applies his business skills as a department manager while the third is about to start a non-profit organization as well as putting his business skills to work in writing grants for his full-time music therapy hospital position.

Obviously, the basic business skills learned in this course segment can be useful beyond starting a private practice. Another application could be program development in agencies, institutions, or organizations, which requires a similar set of skills, a step-by-step process, and proposal outline. However, while this five-week business course segment demonstrated its value as a bridge to the job market, additional pertinent information related to immediate employment, competitive salaries, job satisfaction, and occupation retention of alumni in the field of music therapy and other healthcare professions is needed.

As for this course segment, a more in-depth collaboration with the College of Business is planned. In the future, business students could be involved in implementing the music therapy business plans with alumni. Additional ideas for cross-campus collaborations are discussed. Yet in its infancy, this business course segment is a starting point. In the future, it might be possible to design an entire business course for music therapy graduate students including advanced topics such as management, marketing, customer behavior, and law and ethics. For example, the music therapy graduate program at the Queens University of Charlotte in North Carolina offered a 12-plus hours business concentration taught by the faculty of the McColl School of Business in 2015 (R. Engen, personal communication, December 16, 2016). Nonetheless, there is also an array of short-term business courses offered by experienced music therapy entrepreneurs for ongoing education credits that can assist music therapists to enhance their skills and stay abreast with the latest developments and trends in the field. Besides this, there are many valuable Massive Open Online Courses (MOOCs) about various business aspects that can support healthcare providers to learn more about the business aspect needed in their private practices and beyond. Finally, especially as a new entrepreneur, it is essential to have mentorship from experienced colleagues to establish a successful business in today's market that will be sustainable.

Conclusion

The increase in self-employment and private practice in the healthcare business is calling for action on the part of educators, organizations, and ongoing education providers in the healthcare industry, including the field of music therapy. Progress has been made in establishing various courses and successful private practices in the communities. However, students continue to join the workforce with limited knowledge and experiences in business operations and struggle to make a living as therapists while maintaining their own personal well-being. Thus, teaching and developing business skills must continue so that new professionals gain a better understanding of the business aspect of therapy, develop thriving practices while maintaining a healthy work–life balance, as well as making an adequate income that values the therapists' expertise and services provided to individuals, communities, and society at large. As educators preparing students for the workforce, it is vital to stay informed about employment trends to maximize students' success in finding fulfilling career paths—whether as business owners or employees—that allow them to remain in the profession for a lifetime.

Note: I would like to thank students of the University of Louisville for their inventive exploration of starting a music therapy business and all colleagues who contributed to the success of this course segment.

References

American Music Therapy Association (2013). *American Music Therapy Association Professional Competencies*. Retrieved from www.musictherapy.org/about/competencies on 28 November 2016.

American Music Therapy Association (2014). *American Music Therapy Association Code of Ethics*. Retrieved from www.musictherapy.org/about/ethics on 28 November 2016.

American Music Therapy Association (2015). *Scope of Music Therapy Practice*. Retrieved from www.musictherapy.org/about/scope_of_music_therapy_practice on 28 November 2016.

Behnke, C.A. (1996). My viewpoint: A music therapist and sole proprietorship. *Music Therapy Perspectives*, 14, 1, 61–65.

Certification Board for Music Therapists (2016). *The Certification Board for Music Therapists*. Retrieved from www.cbmt.org on 28 November 2016.

Fulton, K. (producer) (2011, September 15). Music Therapists Talk about Self-Care: A Video Interview [video podcast].

Global Business School Network (2013). *Education, Employment & Entrepreneurship: A Snapshot of the Global Job Challenge*. Retrieved from http://c.ymcdn.com/sites/www.gbsnonline.org/resource/collection/0C22350B-578A-4B69-9730-22A37ED43CFC/GBSN_Report_-_Education_Employment_and_Entrepreneurship.pdf on 29 November 2016.

Grodzki, L. (2015). *Building Your Ideal Private Practice: A Guide for Therapists and Other Healing Professionals* (2nd edition). New York: W.W. Norton & Company Ltd.

Guy, J.M. (2005). *A Survey of Music Therapy Business Owners*. Master's Thesis, Western Michigan University. Retrieved from www.themusictherapycenter.com/sites/default/files/images/articles/mtccaBusSurvey.pdf on 28 November 2016.

Kern, P. (producer) (2014a, 14 June). Getting Ready for the Market [Video]. Retrieved from https://youtu.be/h1KVPvxUVbw on 29 November 2016.

Kern, P. (producer) (2014b, 11 December). Fleur de Lis Music Therapy, LLC [Video]. Retrieved from https://youtu.be/8raZB4_J8CE on 4 December 2016.

Kern, P. (producer) (2016, 5 July). Shark Tank #MUTH432 Style [Video]. Retrieved from www.youtube.com/watch?v=HIzpjdCL_mE on 4 December 2016.

Lacy, L.D. and Hadsell, N.A. (2003). Music therapy practice in the Southwestern region of the American Music Therapy Association: Making a living in a dynamic, complex field. *Music Therapy Perspectives*, 21, 2, 110–112.

Palloff, R.M. and Pratt, K. (2013). *Lesson from the Virtual Classroom: The Realities of Online Teaching*. San Francisco, CA: Jossey-Bass.

Pizzi, M. and Guy, J. (eds.) (2015). *Leading the Way—Music Therapy Business of the Future: A Workbook*. Silver Spring, MD: AMTA.

Rambach, R. (2011). Building your own business in early childhood music therapy. *imagine*, 2, 1, 90.

Selingo, J.J. (2013). *College (Un)bound: The Future of Higher Education and What It Means for Students*. Las Vegas, NV: Amazon Publishing.

Sena Moore, K. (2008). *The Therapy Business Blueprint: 7-Step Approach to Starting Your Own Private Practice* (e-book). Retrieved from www.musictherapyebooks.com/vendor/kimberly-sena-moore on 29 November 2016.

Silverman, M.J. and Furman, A.G. (2014). Employment and membership trends in the American Music Therapy Association, 1998–2009. *Music Therapy Perspectives*, 32, 1, 99–108.

Silverman, M.J., Furman, A.G., Schwartzberg, E.T., Leonard, J., Stephens, E. and McKee, R. (2013). Music therapy salaries from 1998–2012: A comparative and descriptive study. *Music Therapy Perspectives*, 31, 4, 181–188.

Tonkinson, S. (2014). *Marketing in Music Therapy: A Survey of Self-Employed Music Therapists to Identify Methods of Marketing Planning, Positioning, Promotion, and Implementation*. Master's Thesis, Arizona State University. Retrieved from https://repository.asu.edu/attachments/134892/content/Tonkinson_asu_0010N_13738.pdf on 29 November 2016.

Udacity (2016). *About Us*. Retrieved from www.udacity.com/us on 29 November 2016.

US Small Business Administration (n.d.) *Build Your Business Plan*. Retrieved from www.sba.gov/tools/business-plan/1 on 5 December 2016.

Wilhelm, K. (2004). Music therapy and private practice: Recommendations on financial viability and marketing. *Music Therapy Perspectives*, 22, 2, 68–83.

Appendix
Assignment #4 with learning outcomes, dues dates, step-by-step description, evaluation rubrics, and peer ratings template

Assignment #4

Build Your Own Business
Individual & Teamwork: Attend and Participate, Gather Information, Connect With Experts, Join the Career Coach
Prepare for Final Exam (Business Plan, Peer Coaching, Video Clip, and Reflective Essay)

Learning Outcomes
By the end of this assignment you will be able to
- understand the basic concepts to build your own business
- collaborate with potential business partners in setting up a music therapy business
- evaluate the music therapy industry and the current climate and trends
- network and learn from experts in the field
- identify your transferable skills and make use of available resources
- use technology and media for marketing, and
- reflect on your qualities and confidence as a potential entrepreneur.

Due Dates
- Week 1 @ 9 AM-5 PM (EST): Attend and participate at the onsite weekend intensive course
- Week 2 @ midnight on Sunday (EST): Summarize findings in your stand-up report post
- Week 3 @ scheduled appointment: Connect with your assigned experts; stand-up report post
- Week 4 @ midnight on Sunday (EST): Join the coaching session; individual blog post and one peer comment
- Week 5 @ midnight on Sunday (EST): Submit your business plan, video clip, and reflective essay

Steps
1. **Weekend Intensive Course: Attend and Participate**
   a. Read Sena Moore (2008).
   b. Prepare your response to the following questions:
      - What are pros and cons of self-employment, especially for newcomers in the field?
      - Which music therapy private businesses capture your attention and why?
      - How would you get started with building your own business?
   c. Review the recommended resources (i.e., audio podcasts, reports, articles, and books).

2. **Module 1: Gather Information**
   a. Study current workforce trend analysis and organizational workforce data relevant to your region and state.
   b. Review federal, state, and organization policies that may influence your business.
   c. Search the web for similar music therapy businesses and evaluate their services and products.
   d. Explore related local service providers and pinpoint the gaps and needs of your community.
   e. Identify potential clients that could benefit from your unique services and products.
   f. Re-visit the recommended resources (i.e., audio podcasts, reports, articles, and books) as needed and apply information to your unique business.
   g. Provide a summary of your findings and discussions in the stand-up report on the blog.

Spring 2016 – School of Music
Principles & Practices of MT II

Instructor: Dr. Petra Kern

Assignment #4

3. **Module 2: Connect With Experts**
   a. Inform yourself about your assigned music therapy entrepreneur's business.
   b. Prepare 7-10 questions for your music therapy entrepreneur related to your business plan development.
   c. Meet your music therapy entrepreneur online or at the conference site during the scheduled day and time.
   d. Email your 3-5 questions about funding and reimbursements of your prospective music therapy services to the regional AMTA reimbursement representative.
   e. Listen to the experts' advice and embed what you have learned into your business plan.
   h. Provide a summary of at least five takeaways in the stand-up report on the blog.

4. **Module 3: Join the Career Coach**
   a. Participate lively in the coaching session provided by a career coach of the university.
   b. Use your skills and talents identified during the coaching session for your team's business development.
   c. Consider making an individual appointment at the Career Development Center for additional services.
   d. Post a text-based summary of your individual "aha" moments (200-250 words) on the blog.
   e. Post a text-based comment to one peer's blog entry (150-200 words).

5. **Module 4: Prepare for Final Exam**
   a. Business Plan
      - Use the suggested business plan template of the U.S. Small Business Administration and address each section by including the content items descripted.
      - Embed and cite relevant information you have gathered over the past four weeks.
      - Make sure that you are realistic, conservative with investments, and innovative with your services and products. Ultimately, demonstrate your niche!
   b. Peer Coaching
      - Pitch your business proposal in a 10-minute competitive presentation to business school students.
      - Get their direct feedback and tips to strengthen your business proposal in a peer coaching session.
      - Finalize your business plan and reflect suggested improvements.
   c. Video Clip
      - Select a project theme from iMovie or similar software.
      - Produce a 3-minute high quality video clip (including a jingle or music, images, and text) introducing all components of your business (i.e., who, what, when, where, how, and why) to your potential clients.
      - Be creative and make sure that the talents and ideas of all team members are included.
      - Export the movie as MPEG-4 (max. 100 MB).
   d. Reflective Essay
      - Read Grodzki (2015).
      - Write an individual reflective essay addressing the following guiding questions:
         - Which of Grodzki's strategies and ideas resonated most with you?
         - What surprising facts did you find in the text?
         - Which qualities and confidence level do you bring to building your own business?
         - In conclusion, is building your own business something you wish to pursue?
   e. Submit your complete Business Plan, Video Clip, and Reflective Essay along with your peer ratings by Sunday @midnight.

Spring 2016 – School of Music
Principles & Practices of MT II

Instructor: Dr. Petra Kern

Assignment #4

Build Your Own Business
Evaluation Rubrics

STUDENT NAME: DATE:

TEAM MEMBERS:

Assignments	Points	Earned
Attend and Participate (individual student)	10	
❏ Attended the Weekend Intensive Course		
❏ Participated in the discussions and activities by asking questions, making informed comments, and sharing examples and ideas		
Gather Information (student team)	10	
❏ Identified and reflected workforce trends, federal/state/organizational policies, successful music therapy business, community needs and potential clients in the stand-up report		
Connect With Experts (student team)	10	
❏ Prepared relevant questions for experts (i.e., entrepreneur and reimbursement representative)		
❏ Summarized at least five takeaways from expert contacts in the stand-up report		
Join the Career Coach (individual student)	10	
❏ Posted a personal "aha" moment (200-250 words)		
❏ Posted one insightful comment to a peer (150-200 words)		
Prepare for Final Exam		
Business Plan (student team)	20	
❏ Addressed all ten components of the business plan		
❏ Delivered content quality, comprehension, and accuracy (i.e., resources, descriptions, numbers)		
❏ Demonstrated innovation and forward thinking		
Peer Coaching (student team)	10	
❏ Pitched business proposal in a convincing way		
❏ Revised business plan		
Video Clip (student team)	10	
❏ Targeted potential clients addressing who, what, when, where, how, and why		
❏ Produced high quality video file with jingle/music, images, and text, and within time and size limit		
Reflective Essay (individual student)	10	
❏ Reflected the four guiding questions		
❏ Well organized (i.e., layout, formatting) and written (i.e., language, grammar, punctuation)		
Peer Ratings (individual student)	10	
❏ Rate the performance of your team members (template). Think of your peers' reliability, participation, and contributions to Assignment #4		
Total	100	

UNIVERSITY OF LOUISVILLE

Spring 2016 – School of Music
Principles & Practices of MT II

Instructor: Dr. Petra Kern

Assignment #4

Build Your Own Business
Template for Peer Ratings

STUDENT NAME: DATE:

TEAM MEMBERS:

Think of your peers' reliability, participation, and contributions to Assignment #4.

Name of Student	Poor	Needs Improvement	Acceptable	Excellent
	0	1	3	5

CHAPTER 7

Creative Arts Therapies and Business in the USA
Perspectives and Perception
Rebecca Zarate

Introduction

Learning how to navigate any business environment is difficult, but as an American creative arts therapist, there are different layers to consider to that of our international counterparts. First, how the meaning of 'arts' is negotiated through channels of politics, economics and social norms deeply affects how we are 'seen' in the community. Second, we need to consider the economic impact of this as it relates to how creative arts therapists are trained, and their experiences of how they are utilised and/or underutilised in employment within the communities they work in. These two aspects overarch discussion on the business and economic identity of creative arts therapists in the USA. In this chapter I discuss and critique my experience as a music therapist, educator and researcher as it relates to the profession's economic identity, within the context of business and leadership roles I have fulfilled. I also share information gathered from conversations with ten creative arts therapists from a variety of American states with differing business and leadership backgrounds. I offer a collaborative community approach of learning and leadership influenced by Etienne Wenger's work as a way of challenging and solving the larger socio-political issues we face that impact our economy as creative arts therapists.

The production, consumption and transfer of arts therapies in business in communities

There are a number of accessible pathways for creative arts therapists to enter into the business arena. Many begin from foundations of private practice, home-based or rented office-based studio work, or while maintaining a 'day job' in or outside of their field of expertise. The typical business models that are being used during these initial stages of setting up a business are 'Doing Business As' (DBA), which involves sole proprietorships; Limited Liability Companies (LLCs); incorporated businesses, otherwise known as corporations; and finally, the non-clinical consultations, wellness 'therapeutic' services, such as recreation-based workshops. The types of services generally provided are clinical, including single sessions, group sessions, family sessions and psycho-education models.

Another appropriate but less popular route to take is to form a not-for-profit business, or non-profit service, otherwise known by their code of 501c. Many fall under 501c3 or 501c4 because these codes show the public that they are a tax-deductible organisation and can accept donations. It is less popular because it involves a lot more paperwork, effort and other business formalities than the aforementioned. As with all business ventures, the major need is for capital, hard cash, in order to support the initial building years.

Service need and service production: confronting a dilemma

These services generally take years to develop, and require many hours of building clientele and contacts before an individual will make the leap over into full-time business operations. This is the major dilemma and area of tension for many creative arts therapists interested in branching out alone in business. The unpredictability of business coupled with the need to generate financial stability is a real and practical concern. It causes a number of conflicts, and sometimes confusion, between service need and service production. The nuanced details about relationships between which business model to choose and what population to serve are important, but less known in the creative arts therapies community. Choosing a business model that will generate a solid customer relationship management model (CRM) that includes customer satisfaction, customer loyalty, customer tenure and business performance is one of the key areas I noticed work well, but that takes time to think about, learn and to really get to know the community layers and attitudes towards arts and heath.

One key component to achieving this is to understand attitudinal loyalty and behaviour loyalty of customers and staff. According to Buttel, 'attitudinal loyalty is measured by reference to components of attitude such as beliefs, feelings, and purchasing intention. Those customers who have a stronger preference for, involvement in, or commitment to a supplier are the more loyal in attitudinal terms' (2010, p.45). For creative arts therapies, an example of this is when the public experience creative arts therapies in action, in some form of performance-based or demonstration-based promotion, and this can be used as a marketing tool. As creative arts therapists we have disciplinary knowledge, and this suggestion would make sense to many readers because of that. We have yet to find pathways into an interdisciplinary model of knowledge that includes the field of leadership and business. When there is a tracking method, such as the one outlined here, where we can track the above-mentioned marketing plan, it is easier to use the data to screen for attitude and behaviour patterns of consumption and production. This then helps us to build a business that is in touch with the population need we are serving and the business model that will deliver it.

Considering cross-cultural tensions

The role of insurance in shaping creative arts business practice in America

It is important to consider the cross-cultural context of leadership within our economy, in terms of a process-driven 'product' of creative arts therapies. This means we are identified with, and operate from, a 'short-term orientation characterised by demands for immediate results and a low propensity to save' (Pierce & Newstrom 2008, p.217). In the USA, clinicians in business are required to have personal and company liability insurance *and* also need some form of health insurance. This puts a great deal of financial strain on a small business. According to the US Department of Health and

Human Services (DHHS) report from 2015 to 2016, the average monthly range for premium for insurance was USD $396–$502 for individuals in full-time employment with benefit plans (DHHS 2016, p.9) and an average range of $667–$1403 for family coverage (Merhar 2016). Access to health insurance could be a real barrier to business development for a creative arts therapist. This is why seeking employment within institutions is often a favourable option, as liability and health insurance are covered and offered as part of the employment package with choices that are adaptable for family needs.

The cost of doing business in arts-friendly communities in America

Another cross-cultural tension is seen in the barriers presented to renting appropriate therapy space. Communities that are creative arts therapy-friendly tend to be in geographic areas where offices are expensive to rent, and generally not equipped to satisfy the needs for the kind of arts-based work involved in creative arts therapy sessions. Certain individuals across the country have grouped together to create cooperative practices that are either individual and separate but share rent, or operate under a business name and split workload and profits for a percentage based on ownership of the business and titles. This may be a model that other professionals are also following internationally.

The social consumption of arts therapies in America and the impact of this on licensing

The American public generally consumes creative arts therapies via socially focused services, due to a host of challenges and opportunities that support or diffuse clinically focused practice on a state-by-state case. The United States has legislature that requires any master's-level clinician wanting to practise, or be hired to do clinical work, to have a current state license. This means that certain professions are considered within a field to be valued as 'clinical'. Creative arts and clinical practice does not fit into the traditional dominant narrative of scientific evidence-based practice. Unfortunately, the creative arts therapies are one of those groups that is an outlier to that current social-medical norm. Furthermore, out of the 50 states, there is only one that has an indigenous Creative Arts Therapies License, the LCAT, in New York. Hilary Clinton supported the passage of the bill which came into effect in 2006, an important political fact to consider at this particular moment in time. The other states do not recognise the creative arts therapies as billable clinical practice, although some have passed bills that license specific fields. There has been a need for creativity to adjust, align and lobby to be a part of a license that includes creative arts therapies. An example would be the Massachusetts license which is called the Licensed Massachusetts Counselor of Mental Health, LMCH. No state license is transferable between states, which causes disparity and inequity in the employment–practice relationship.

Health insurance companies are bountiful in the USA, and also an imbedded vital economic consideration for individuals as they dictate the kind of healthcare American citizens receive. Insurance companies require state licences for clinical services to be provided to their members. Without licensure, a creative arts therapist is limited to the types of service they can charge for, and are automatically eliminated from the general public eye and expectation of what is available for healthcare. There is also an imbedded dynamic and explicit interest between health insurance companies and pharmaceutical companies, otherwise known as 'Big Pharma'. Big Pharma is responsible for what is marketed and pushed onto the public in specific communities and demographics, creating a vacuum of access to and choice of a complete range of adequate and appropriate treatments. These are very real impediments for creative arts therapists who have earned master's-level degrees in order to meet state legislation requirements. For the clinician who is interested in beginning a private practice, and who has vast experience with a clinical population who is not marketed by Big Pharma, it becomes economically non-viable. An example of this would be an experienced creative arts therapist interested in beginning a private practice to provide service in an area of expertise in the community, such as complex trauma. Due to this specific approach to mental health not supported by the Big Pharma – insurance – medical field stream, access to such a service cannot be gained easily, or at all, by those who may need and respond best to this approach. Consumption cannot be defined appropriately or accordingly, because of this kind of barrier to the public.

A community-based approach to health-care in America

Given that creative arts therapies (CAT) are literally the outliers of a health system that is serving the few and not the many, and as a movement towards the affordable healthcare act moves closer to reality, there could be opportunities to create a space for producing and consuming creative arts therapies as part of this community-based approach to healthcare.

This does, however, present the profession with both disciplinary and interdisciplinary dilemmas of how to forge ahead with identity as each field matures and decides which direction to go in: to branch off, such as art therapy is beginning to do, and/or to continue to develop a collaborative identity through operations such as the National Coalition of the Creative Arts Therapies Associations (NCCATA). Transferring the practice of creative arts therapies is, as one can imagine, no easy task, given the political environment of healthcare in America. The ways in which it is occurring outside of major CAT-friendly cities, like New York City, is by way of survival, knowledge of the power of the work, and sheer passion to serve communities. There is a strong disciplinary knowledge that people respond to in creative arts therapies clinical practice. In response to identifying the need to transfer this knowledge to the larger community, the NCCATA past president shared that in the last four years, 'all [professions in the coalition] worked hard at getting out more into the public view' (personal communication, 12 September 2016). This is a testament to the commitment to lobbying and determination to move the profession forward by each of the professional organisations.

Another way of approaching licensing issues in America

A reprieve from the intense political healthcare climate of state licensure is that each profession that falls under the canopy of CAT (art, dance/movement, drama, music, and poetry) has its own way of legitimising specific scope of practice through its professional organisations and certifying body. These board certifications are transferable across states, which makes employment and economic movement accessible. One caveat to that is that within music therapy the certification is considered equal for baccalaureate and master's-level training. It is different to its counterpart fields that have a tiered system of evaluation that correlates with scope of practice. How this is transferred into the community certainly affects how the public consumes the services because there is a wide variety of practice, which shapes perception. It is causing a confused transfer of what music therapy is, and in the wider scheme of things, contributes towards confusion about CAT. As a result of this landscape, creative arts therapists who are interested in branching out into their own business endeavours must face this reality, and find a philosophical, ethical and practical way to succeed. A colleague who is a music psychotherapist, educator and business owner shared that his experience of non-transferable licensure makes it difficult to find the right therapist for the specific contract as well as being able to practise individually. But he also felt lucky to have the MT-BC (Music Therapy – Board Certified). Another colleague who is an arts therapist in management and consulting shared:

> A very specific challenge that I have faced as a LCAT in New York was when I moved to Rhode Island the license did not exist in Rhode Island.

This kind of struggle sets up hierarchical dynamics in the workplace. Some colleagues shared comments such as an inability to find full-time work and its impact on professional identity, morale, livelihood and access:

> Finding full-time work as a music therapist, not as a music therapist/what-else-do-I-have-to-do-to-have-a-full-time-job-here (acknowledging that I am one of the lucky ones who can actually have full-time work based, at least in substantial part, around being a music therapist).

> Having to fight my way in to being an 'official' member of a patient's treatment team.

> In the culture of music therapy in California it's very rare that a music therapist has a full-time gig. You piece together work or you piece together contracts unless you are lucky enough to work for the state. Everyone [MTs] I talk to, they would prefer full-time work, because [otherwise] you have to do a lot of driving.

In addition to the CAT discourse, there is also the expressive arts therapies (ExAT) which have developed and matured since their inception at Lesley University 42 years ago. ExAT draws from a theoretical foundation of all of the arts as a means to integrate and transfer as its practice. The international organisation International Expressive Arts Therapies Association (IEATA) has positioned itself in a way that allows for clinical and political flexibility. Co-chairing the European chapter for this organisation was an interesting journey and perspective for me, because I was able to attend to my bi-cultural lens and see where the flexibility in such a position was, as well as where the fluidity of boundaries caused confusion for the profession. I had many conversations about this with my colleagues at Lesley because we combine counselling training, specialisation and ExAT. It continues to push us to think about identity and its relationship to the economy of the creative arts therapies for now and for future generations of clinicians.

A response from art therapy has been to create its own specific and indigenous licensure. It is also the oldest and biggest organisation with the largest membership in the creative arts therapies. The smaller memberships, such as drama and dance, are not in the same situation. The nuances between each field and profession within the creative arts therapies umbrella are part of the complex identity questions and decisions that are made which affect the field's material prosperity.

While the state licensure is limiting, one colleague, who is an art therapist, shared how she was able to find ways into leadership roles because of such nuances between creative arts therapy fields and states:

> I found that New York, specifically the New York City area, has many career options for expressive arts therapists. The field has been well established, there are many universities in the area training new art therapy professionals, and there are so many facilities that understand the value of the profession. I lived and worked as an art therapist in New York for ten years. I was employed at three different hospitals as an art therapist (and as an art therapy supervisor) to provide art therapy. While working at one of these facilities I was able to educate and demonstrate the skills, tools, and benefits of art therapy. I was hired (after working as a consultant for two years) full time in a position as a 'clinical psychologist'. In this capacity

I was able to assist in rebuilding the therapeutic day program in the hospital.

A dance/movement therapist in private practice and in a hospital setting shared:

> I'm working as a psychologist for the state of Rhode Island. My years of experience and training are considered equivalent to that of an MA psychologist. I can continue to facilitate CAT groups within this position. My clinical supervisor is a BC-ATR.

While she shared these opportunities, she also shared her belief that the 'roots [of dance movement therapy] need to be kept as dance'.

Training and transferring the creative arts craft

Training and transfer of the craft is a real political and economic issue in this country. The schools that teach the arts therapies tend to be private (and expensive) universities and colleges, limiting access to the field. Creating access to training programmes in universities and colleges beyond the private sector is a national need in all the arts therapies in order to shape a diverse and inclusive field.

As highlighted before, music therapy has an undergraduate entry level and the same board certificate for both undergraduate and graduate degrees. Training for each is obviously very different, and more sophisticated as the degrees move up in rank. The services that are provided shape the perception of what music therapy is. Providing a clear and consistent message to the public about what music therapy is facing can be difficult. This is a professional issue that is at the forefront of a national movement and dialogue within the AMTA. A music therapy colleague from Florida described the local situation:

> A major challenge is the MT-BC. The perception of music therapy [in Florida] is that it is activity-based work. I had to lean on the fact I had mental health counselling training to give it that weight. Whenever I don't, particularly because I work with children, it becomes music time and not therapy. The perception is that it is recreational, fun, happy times. I always have to bring in the mental health counselling. I tried to get a music therapist to come when

my son was in the hospital. Called the person in charge of the programme. It was clear that there was a behavioural foundation and the music therapist had a pre-arranged schedule. This hinders the perception of music therapy.

A colleague who has her own business from Utah shared this information:

> Utah is not willing to license music therapy. The perception is often that music therapy is a 'fun activity' and when there is a change needed, they are not prepared to have a music therapist in who is doing clinical work. I have to work at re-educating the team as to the clinical aspects of music therapy, requesting charting, assessment, team meeting time... Very tough to re-establish what we are. Part of this becomes a challenge when we are looking at entry-level professionals, with little experience, marketing themselves to advanced-level facilities.

In my conversations with colleagues, there was an overarching concern about the balance between training, marketing services and competencies for services. It also showed a need for survival and creativity in an unfriendly and hostile legislative environment for the creative arts therapies. The local dynamics and divides that have intrinsically been created between entry-level and advanced-level music therapists, and overspill of social and professional dynamics were also in the air of the conversations. From both perspectives, however, what has been revealed is that a clearer message of what creative arts therapies (particularly music therapy) are, and why they are valuable, needs to be implemented in the profession's discourse.

A changing landscape

The landscape is changing, however. Recently, the state of California acknowledged music therapy as a viable treatment for autism. I discussed the implications of this on practice and recognition with a music therapy colleague, who is also an autism specialist and clinical director. She agreed that it had made a big impact on the transfer of knowledge about music therapy in this particular population. In 2015, in a meeting I was a part of, the AMTA named this as a major milestone in discourse. As a group, we came up with population-based research agendas to build the same kind of body of knowledge that can be transferred and translated into practice and into the public domain. The recent past-president of NCCATA similarly commented to me recently that 'using research to support assumptions of what it is that we do [can lead us towards] strong economic potential'.

Two paradigms of CAT business

Two main areas have emerged from my interviews with my colleagues. The first is that people who have started and maintained businesses seem to have a prevalent combination of practitioner identity, sense of community and social responsibility, and some form of leadership characteristic or skillset. This was consistent no matter what business model they used, such as non-profit, social enterprise or for-profit models. It was also consistent that the founders were the practitioners faced with the everyday dilemmas about how to design and maintain a flexible business model that would sustain transfer of ownership from generation to generation. The other emergent area was that of autonomy of practice. This was important for those who had a strong practitioner identity and a need for flexibility and liberty of schedule, but did not follow a specific business model other than a private-practice, for-profit, model.

Social responsibility, practice and community: case examples

Cecile Reve, ExAT, LMHC, is the founder and CEO of ARTrelief in Massachusetts, and began the business eight years ago. She described how she valued having flexibility to pursue running her own business which had socially conscious values and a person/human-centred focus. She spoke of a 'generally positive perception locally/nationally [of ExAT] because we are in an era where people seek alternatives to medical model treatment'. While this is generally an agreed-upon perspective, it is not translating into the healthcare economic market just yet. There is still a disparity between supply and demand. It also questions the relationship between the market economy and political economy of clinical treatment. In a market economy, the consumer is driving the product, yet when the product is placed upon the consumer (as with the situation here in the USA with certain models and medication), other types of services such as creative arts therapies are squeezed out of the conversation. Cecile's area of expertise and experience does suggest that having the choice and the liberty of what and how services are provided is beneficial for overall perception and education.

Farmer and colleagues (2013) refer to the term 'social suffering', a concept developed by Kleinman, Das and Lock (1997), as a way to enter into a candid philosophical critique on the impact of social forces in healthcare. They describe social suffering as a way to 'account for the forms of social violence that constitute inequity' (Farmer et al. 2013, p.30). From the authors' perspectives, social suffering looks at what political, economic and institutional power does to people, and how these forms of power themselves influence responses to social problems:

> The term also encompasses the interpersonal experience of suffering, the experience of chronic illness, and the ways in which society and its institutions unintentionally exacerbate social and health problems. The concept of social suffering addresses the intersection of medical and social problems—for example, the need for coordination of social and health policies in response to clustering of inner-city violence, substance abuse, depression, and suicide. (p.30)

The theory of 'structural violence' developed by Paul Farmer fits within the concept of social suffering and addresses, as he describes, the 'roots of global health inequities…in particular, connecting poverty and ill health within structured processes that limit choices due to racism, sexism, and political violence' (Farmer *et al.* 2013, p.30).

Diana Feldman, founder and director of ENACT, NYC, a non-profit creative arts business that has been operating for 28 years, holds a social justice value that also supports a call to action based on the above description of social suffering and structural violence. She commented that:

> Getting into schools is including kids who may not be able to afford therapy. Providing access. So much complex trauma from living in poverty. Finally, the New York school system is providing clinics and programs in the schools so kids can have access. We have begun training social workers who need to engage with kids and the community.

A colleague working within the hospital psychiatric and mental health system discussed transfer of consultant role into director role to expand services for patients, and provide a new economy for creative arts therapists in the area:

> As a supervisor, I have helped to introduce and create an expressive arts therapy program at this hospital that provides evening and weekend groups to the patients. We have added four creative arts therapist consultants to our department.

Leadership identity and practitioner identity: case examples

Historical context as it related to profession maturity and identity development repeatedly came up in conversations with several colleagues.

From the drama therapy perspective:

> I think I am still in business because I worked out what worked for me. I don't follow how you are supposed to run a traditional non-profit. I am a practitioner first. I developed the method in drama therapy. ENACT is a method. In order to get the method out I had to create a business.

From the dance/movement perspective:

> There was no licensure track when I started, and there wasn't a name for dance-movement therapy… The [ongoing] lack of understanding is preventing primary therapy treatment…roots still must be in dance.

For these leader-practitioners, the sense of social need and knowledge of what they had to offer came through powerfully. Without assuming that three individuals represent all business owners in creative arts therapists, as one who has been in business and leadership positions, I can certainly identify with the drive for creating opportunities and spaces for addressing bigger picture issues and access for services and employment.

From this feedback, it became clear that a theme between method and brand was prevalent, indicating deep-rooted philosophical and ideological foundations of art-form, and arts as therapy. Furthermore, ethical issues were identified as important and pertinent to practice. For example, a colleague from Utah shared:

> My business serves adolescents, adults in recovery, some specialty groups (Vets [veterans], epilepsy) and adult and paediatric hospices. We have several subcontractors and music and art therapy interns. We are a small LLC, no debt, and are committed to high-quality service and paying our subcontractors well. I consider myself a music-centred music therapist; my master's focused on music-centred psychotherapy. My role in the practice is therapist, internship director, and I am responsible for most administrative duties as well; invoicing, payroll, program development, website…we do use a marketing specialist right now in order to give me more time to focus on clinical work and the interns.

As well as:

> My staff always knew I couldn't do this work if I didn't have 100 per cent integrity.

It is logical that creative arts therapists in business and leadership would have a clear philosophical foundation to approaching any kind of business idea as well as considering ethical issues surrounding the economics of that idea. The concern still remains as to how seriously each of the art forms are taken as a clinical tool for healing. Furthermore, within this environment, the tensions that clinical business owners face regarding maintaining values and ethics stirs up an interesting and tough conversation, particularly in regard to gaining contracts, and methods of generating business. (For more information pertaining to ethics refer to Chapter 5 in this book.) Cecile from ARTrelief also discussed how in the private, social enterprise environment, the values of community and group are engaged in different ways internationally. She shared that:

> Internationally, Canada is very much in alliance with expressive arts therapy. Europeans seem more sceptical of a non-established profession and our field isn't established due to lack of supporting research and public policies. More group-oriented cultures (e.g. South America, Caribbean, Africa, Native American…) are more in alignment with our values and sometimes trust our model more than the medical one.

It began with a meeting...

Many times we hear business owners across all sectors tell how an idea was drawn on a napkin, or happened as part of an interview. My perspective on this is that the emergence of an idea was a creative act of synergy between people in context that brought a phenomenon to life which was already there. The stories that I heard were that 'It came organically in a [practice-based] conversation', 'I/we needed to do something for the community, because there is a lack of service/knowledge.' For some important reason, unbeknown to the naked eye, there was an idea borne out of that encounter. Here are some thoughts from colleagues who had found a 'hole in the market' organically:

> I found a need for music psychotherapy services with those who were diagnosed with dementia after a conversation with my supervisor who is now my colleague, and I began to contract out my services, and then expand into other areas locally, and now I have some contracts in other states.
>
> NCCATA started in the 1970s to have a bigger public presence for getting the public to know about it.
>
> This endeavour helped me grow as a professional and I was given the opportunity to supervise the department of psychology including nine master's-level clinicians including LMHC, ATR, MT and DMT as well as ten behaviour specialists.

My personal experience

In my own experience, I have been involved in community-based work for over 20 years in a variety of arts-based, clinical and leadership capacities. I took an administrative position at 25 years old, without official training, but with a decent amount of clinical and community experience, vision and potential to develop solid leadership skills. I initiated the conversation with my then boss, after all my peers and others had turned down the position! I was also lucky enough to receive a work visa, which is beyond the scope of this chapter, but relevant to the larger conversation of employment and diversity in the field. I received executive director training to support building larger projects and teams. Learning how to navigate the dynamics of the hospital industry in all its complexities was challenging.

However, the vision and mission to expand the work to provide access to treatment for the patients, and training/education for psychologists, social workers and doctors, was too important for me to not do. I harnessed my abilities for both administrative and creative, 'out of the box' thinking which proved to be an asset in a very concrete and numbers-driven environment. If it was not the right time for the team to understand a *creative* idea – for example, painting soft colours and clouds in the 'quiet room' for traumatised children – I would use the legislation from the governing bodies as well as my vision to reframe. In some cases, I was able to find a way to get projects done, and in other cases, I could not, until these 'ideas' were being required from the same governing bodies based on new research coming through the pipeline.

Meanwhile, I tried out private practice, which grew fast and was exciting, but I couldn't manage the cash-flow on my own, because I was following a DBA model, and was taken by surprise. I needed to balance out percentages of the practice that were insurance reimbursements, private payers, contracts, and was also offered an opportunity to make room for pro bono work. In that time, I found a community of scholars, clinicians and conference organisers who were into trying out an idea of bringing all the arts therapies together to form an Expressive Therapies Summit in NYC, which worked, and although I left the committee to finish my PhD, it is still bringing therapists together and has become a part of the national arts therapies conference circuit and is gaining some traction internationally.

We had our usual holiday lunch together, and she told me she was selling the business...

The story continues with me taking over a business that I was practising in as a music psychotherapist and programme coordinator at the time. It was the most stressful and most rewarding business project that I have taken on so far. It was a mid-sized business, for-profit, LLC private music school. This was not in New York, and so I faced the issue of navigating how I was going to continue to work clinically without a state licence, and what that meant ethically for my private practice and moving my clients over a state line. I also had to contend with building up an already small but established music therapy programme. At the same time, I was trying to pay back an enormous loan, parallel to accruing student loans from my doctoral training. The guilt of potentially losing my home for a business venture was palpable. In a moment of either altered state or clarity, or both, I realised that I was exactly where I needed to be. Once this happened, I was able to focus on looking at this particular school's place in the community, its cash-flow, its reputation, and what was needed. It was housed in a centre for the arts, and there were many vibrant businesses that were wonderful, and also competition! My stance was that arts therapies and arts education was vital for this particular community and coming together in a consortium using a community learning model and a multiple intelligences model to strategise made good business sense for all of us. We could stay 'separate yet related', to use the analogy from attachment theory.

It takes a village-community, relationships and empowerment

In 2011 we launched the consortium which offered a series of open houses and community-based work to expose and educate about arts in education and creative arts therapies. It was successful in generating business and interest, as well as getting the macro- and micro-levels of exposure out into the community. The east side of town needed to know about what we were doing as well as the west side of town. If successful, it would also dismantle underlying ethnic and class divides and bring people together. It also mattered how we business owners communicated and treated each other. Here are some thoughts from my notes on this project:

> There is never time to sit with colleagues when you own and manage a business. It has a strange dynamic of never alone because you are always networking or dealing with people in a variety of contexts, but you are isolated in that you do not have time to resource and reflect with colleagues on the larger social and economic problems you are all facing in a community.

This consortium model allowed for collaborative decision-making. It was also a sign that I had evolved in my leadership capacity and had found a place to apply my love of learning theories for social action and put that into practice. Offering free services and reaching out to the community in crises was another way of working from the philanthropy prong of the business, and from my philosophy towards access to services for all.

When super-storm Sandy hit land, the centre was shut down, flooded, and my colleagues who had businesses on the first floor had lost everything: large corporate restaurants to small, one-person-owned DBAs. I had staff and their families who were living in the shelters. My apartment building, a 17-floor high-rise, had lost all water, heat and electric, and stairs were the only way to leave and enter. My husband and I, as many of us in the community able to do so, were on the building delivery team to take food, water and blankets for those who could not use the stairs. First thing in the mornings, we would do our building delivery assignments and then check in with friends and colleagues in the business community. Some colleagues had water and heat back before others, and every day we all found a way to meet and figure out who needed showers, picking up from the shelter, and hot food and clean clothes. I believe that it was the consortium that brought that level of companionship and compassion to the business environment at the centre, which helped in the emotional and economic healing from super-storm Sandy. Moreover, the importance of community in business and leadership, for me, was epitomised when a dear colleague rallied students to provide the music school community staff and faculty families with blankets, socks and flashlights in the shelters. The AMTA did a national rally to compose a set list of songs for the makeshift kitchens we were creating so that we could provide some comfort and normality for each other. To this day, the gratitude that I feel about that moment in time for the compassionate reciprocity and help I received, and the help that, as a business, I was able to provide for the families, is visceral. Beyond the strategic planning, budget, research agenda and administrative items is ethical practice and quality service, and most of all, advocacy, people and relationships. Community epistemology in my work is at the heart of what I currently consider a 'practice of leadership'. I teach my students about practising academic humility and a willingness to sit with and embrace multiplicity.

The themes of my story mirror the challenges and opportunities that my creative arts therapist colleagues have shared and face here in the States.

Community ventures

There is an entrepreneurial-creative spirit characteristic that comes with being able to tolerate the risk and reward rollercoaster of business and management in creative arts therapies. I have certainly brought tough lessons learned along the way, as well as sheer delightfulness of a sense of purpose. In the last several years, I have become involved in a new community venture.

I had not experienced working for or designing a non-profit until recently with Butterfly Music, a registered 4013c (a specific and most popular type of not-for-profit business model), and also in my current role at Lesley University, a non-profit, private university. I have returned to working in larger systems and organisations, with an evolved and deepened set of skills. With Butterfly, it began with a meeting with the director, Sandi Hammond. She was reaching out to explore interest in the area of creating support through music education, vocal education and music therapy for gender issues, for women, and for the transgender community. After a thoughtful and enthusiastic conversation, we began to work together as part of a core group with a variety of expertise to begin to assist Sandi to structure and build a non-profit that would support an interdisciplinary model of vocal education for transgender people so that educational, psychological and physical needs were being met. This came out of an organic need in the community in her voice lessons. In practice, we were beginning to see that the need for a combined set of skills was vital due to the lack of support for transgender people in the community, and the powerful impact singing was having on the individuals and chorus group as a whole community. A series of several workshops has taken place since then where we have offered vocal training as part of a three-pronged approach we have named 'vocal knowledge'. This approach enlists expertise from music (vocal) educators and performers, music therapists, and speech pathologists within an arts-based enquiry model.

While it is a lot of fun to collaborate with other colleagues from other disciplines, it has also meant that we have been able to 'spread the wealth' of a variety of our different 'currencies' locally and globally, which we bring to the table and move into an interdisciplinary model for this particular organisation model. The need for flexibility within an organisation structure also came up in my conversations, and knowing how to navigate that space can be tricky without the education, training or experience. Forging a community of expertise is essential because it could mean the difference between success and going bust. Maybe the same philosophy is needed within the creative arts therapies business conversation?

Is there a need for business training or mentoring communities?

Although I cannot represent the whole community on this topic, there seems to be a pattern of those who have gone into business in the last 35 years having succeeded (in part, or possibly fully) because they sort out some form of expanded knowledge around business. This has manifested in either another degree in business and management, training and new knowledge of business, or other personal or professional resources in their circles to support the plan. Wenger-Trayner et al. (2014) describe the thought behind what they call 'a model of convening roles' as part of a theory of transformational and critical learning. They comment that 'crossing the boundaries that separate people who do related work gives them a new sense of their field of action. Such transformations of identity happen over time, but it ends up driving thought and behavior across situations' (Wenger-Trayner et al. 2014, p.143).

For example, I looked to alternative knowledge paths to feel more confident in what I was doing in business. I took a summer intensive course at New York University (using my accrued credits from teaching and supervising). It was called 'How to start your own business on a shoestring'. I still have my notes from that course, because it was so valuable, and a good way to begin to look at what I was able to do on my own and what other resources I needed before I launched my first business in music therapy and community wellness. In my conversation with the past chair of NCCATA, she reflected that historically, creative arts therapies are a practice-based profession with no administrative or business foundations. She also shared that, 'In order to progress, the only option would be to move into administration. People got into administrative positions without any managerial training. Some were very good at it and some were not.'

The function of leadership has not traditionally been in curriculum or training models of creative arts therapies until very recently. It has only been experienced inadvertently through clinical supervision. Yet, there are creative arts therapists in the profession who are interested, and may not have the skills, but do have the characteristics, epistemology and worldview that could be aligned for leadership and business roles. On the other hand, it seems that there is a need for more full-time positions that do not require the kind of skillset and resources needed to operate a business. It would be interesting to explore this relationship further. The responsibility, education and training that is needed to run an organisation is plentiful, and may have a purpose inside or outside of curriculum within local and national communities through identifying a group of mentors to support and train those interested. I certainly infuse my experience into my teaching and advising of my MA and PhD students, but do not currently provide any explicit business or managerial training within the curriculum.

> When you run an organisation, all people care about is outcomes. Evidence-based literature, then you cannot get funding. You are now a researcher. Then you need the money.
>
> I think consistently, the magic of the program, once you see it, they are pretty blown away by it. You're a politician, a lobbyist, a practitioner, and then you have to navigate. Constantly watch the competition. You're training people at night. We have extensive training materials. Let's have a look at the quality and ethics. (Diana Feldman, ENACT, personal communication)

Understanding the dynamics and language of business and management is an important and key feature of being able to support oneself and the business. There is certainly a need for training, and Petra Kern explores this topic further in Chapter 6 of this book.

I believe this training needs to happen in partnership with all stakeholders: educators, clinicians and business owners who have all succeeded in seeking knowledge and training and have the experience to share. One of the business owners I spoke with mentioned that he would have liked to have been given at least leadership resources in his training, or exposure somehow to the world of business and how it related to clinical business. Finding the holes in the market organically would then be identified as strategic assessments of need, and business plan and model development could be useful to shape access to the larger community using the concepts and methods discussed. It could also be beneficial to view the creative arts therapies field from a micro-economics perspective: using models that reflect efficiency of exchange of 'product' to explore, as Pindyck and Rubinfeld suggest, 'If trade is beneficial, which trades can occur? Which of those trades will allocate goods efficiently among customers? How much better off will consumers then be?' (2009, p.591). Using methods that represent various distributions of resources, such as the 'Edgeworth box', to experiment with all possible allocations of goods and services in creative arts therapies could be a relevant economic idea. As they describe, 'all possible allocations of either two goods between two people or of two inputs between two production processes' (2009, p.591) can be explored as a way to gain a data-driven sense of where, globally, the creative arts therapies can find a solid sustainable economic strategy.

Moving forward

I asked my colleagues what they felt was needed in their field to move the creative arts therapies profession forward towards more opportunities for business, employment and services. The general opinion anchored around wanting to see the profession grow as a result of stronger strategies towards education and lobbying. This included changing the entry-level criteria for music therapy to minimise confusion, finding ways into legislature that support indigenous licensing, and using research to support legislation and licensing change. Offering a community-based model of learning in order to tackle these larger social problems could be the way to move ahead in and between each of the arts therapies field. At the very least, the conversation has begun and by offering this snapshot of internal economic dynamics of creative arts therapies in the USA, I hope that more conversations and movement in this area will occur.

Thank you to the colleagues who generously gave their time to talk with me: their expertise, experience and willingness to pass along knowledge about this complicated landscape is invaluable for shaping our economic discourse.

References

Buttel, F. (2010). *Customer Relationship Management: Concepts and Technologies* (2nd edition). Oxford: Elsevier Ltd.

DHHS (2016). *Marketplace Premiums after Shopping, Switching, and Premium Tax Credits, 2015–0216.* ASPE. Retrieved from https://aspe.hhs.gov/pdf-report/marketplace-premiums-after-shopping-switching-and-premium-tax-credits-2015-2016 on 29 November 2016.

Farmer, P., Kleinman, A., Kim, J. and Basilico, M. (2013). *Reimagining Global Health: An Introduction.* Berkeley, CA: University of California Press.

Kleinman, A., Das, V. and Lock, M. (eds) (1997). *Social Suffering.* Oakland, CA: University of California Press.

Merhar, C. (2016). *Small Business Employee Benefits and HR Blog: FAQ – How Much Does Individual Healthcare Cost?* Retrieved from www.zanebenefits.com/blog/bid/97380/faq-how-much-does-individual-health-insurance-cost on 29 November 2016.

Pierce, J.L. and Newstrom, J.W. (2008). *Leaders and the Leadership Process: Readings, Self-Assessments and Applications* (6th edition). New York: McGraw-Hill.

Pindyck, R. and Rubinfeld, D.L. (2009). *Microeconomics* (7th edition). Upper Saddle River, NJ: Pearson Prentice Hall.

Wenger-Trayner, E., Fenton-O'Creevy, M., Hutchinson, S., Kubiak, C. and Wenger-Trayner, B. (2014). *Learning in Landscapes of Practice: Boundaries, Identity, and Knowledgeability in Practice-Based Learning.* New York: Routledge.

CHAPTER 8

Case Study: Developing an Arts Therapy Practice

Elaine Matthews Venter

Introduction

I am a recently qualified arts therapist, in private practice in Auckland, New Zealand. This chapter focuses on how I am developing my arts therapy private practice, and arts in the workplace consultancy. The decision to go into private practice rather than search for full-time employment was motivated primarily by my desire to work for myself, and also by my understanding that there are very few arts therapy positions available to arts therapists in medical or mental health institutions in New Zealand. I began my training with an awareness of the shortage of arts therapy positions, but was inspired by a commitment to engage in meaningful, creative, rewarding and socially valuable employment. Online searches for arts therapy positions in hospitals and mental health facilities typically yield negative results, while the need for psychologists, allied health professionals, occupational therapists, dieticians, physiotherapists, speech therapists or support workers remains constant. Despite this, I am aware that some of my colleagues have found employment in education, health and child welfare.

It is commonly known that Whitecliffe College of Arts and Design is currently the only provider of an arts therapy training programme in New Zealand which meets all the requirements for professional registration.

Making effective use of clinical placements to gain experience and build networks

As there are so few mental health facilities and hospitals in New Zealand that provide clients with access to arts therapy, the task of finding clinical placements or internships presented me with a significant challenge. In my search for placement opportunities, I sent requests and information letters to a wide range of organisations such as rehabilitation centres, hospitals, prisons and community mental health organisations. Those institutions that responded positively, and which offered placements, provided a wealth of experience, as well as valuable networking opportunities. My placements enabled me to practice skills in group and individual arts therapy, to develop a sense of the client populations I felt most drawn to working with, and to form an idea of the potential areas of future specialisation.

Regular supervision, as well as daily entries into a visual journal, facilitated an authentic awareness of my creative, physical and emotional responses to the placement experiences. Journaling also provided me with valuable insight into my countertransference in relation to clinical environments and client populations. It was important to trust these insights, and to pay attention to the content and themes that appeared in my art, and to bring these to supervision. I found that it was equally important to maintain an awareness of my physical responses to workplace environments, and to the groups and individual clients I interacted with. Feelings of exhaustion, emotional strain, muscle tension, headaches, and feelings of being overwhelmed would be calls to pay more attention to my own wellbeing. I was advised by my supervisor to make the time to engage in effective self-care strategies such as attending regular therapy. Engaging in creative and physical activities which enhanced my enjoyment and relaxation also became a vital practice, which I continue now that I am in private practice.

Exploring priorities

Before starting off in private practice, it was necessary to explore my priorities, and to build a picture of the path I hope to follow as my career evolves. Here the process of regular creative journaling is helpful. As a first step to creating an idea of how I hoped my life and career to evolve, I adapted the solution-focused therapy directive, 'the Miracle Question' (de Shazer 1988), to suit my purposes. This activity helped me to imagine, and to visualise an ideal scenario, in finding clarification with regard to my professional requirements as an arts therapist, and as an artist, as well as my personal needs as a parent, and as a partner in a relationship. To gain further self-insight, and to establish how I planned to develop an identity as an arts therapist, I asked myself four simple but important questions: who, where, what and how. Consideration of these questions was an exercise in clarification, and the answers provided entry points into understanding what I wanted from my career.

Who?

I am comfortable working with a wide range of people, with men, women and children across the life span, and in group settings. The client populations I find particularly meaningful to work with include immigrants, and those in recovery from trauma and substance abuse. I also enjoy facilitating arts events in workplaces and organisations. These events focus on enhancing communication skills and creative thinking, reducing work-related stress, building team identity, and encouraging happiness, enthusiasm and wellbeing. Another area that I find particularly rewarding is eco-art therapy, which involves using natural materials found in the natural environment, as it is a powerful way to enhance recovery, and a sense of connection and belonging.

Where?

This question is answered by taking my personality, lifestyle, location, and the needs of my young family into consideration. I appreciate the flexibility of working in private practice, and being contracted to organisations or workplaces to run arts therapy groups. I enjoy working independently, rather than being employed full time in an institution. I prefer to work close to my home, rather than to travel long distances, and have therefore chosen to hire a studio and practice room in a local community centre that is in close proximity to my home.

What?

As a visual artist, with an MA in Fine Art, the question of 'what' might seem self-evident, but the multimodal nature of my training provided an awareness of the rich diversity and potential for healing that can be offered when incorporating the natural environment, movement, mindfulness, and a more embodied, integrated therapeutic approach with my primary modality, visual arts therapy.

How?

Once I had gained an understanding of my priorities and requirements, I was ready to begin the process of establishing and running an arts therapy private practice and arts in the workplace consultancy. The question of 'how' is essentially the focus of this chapter.

Registering a business

My very first steps were to decide upon a business name, and to register it with the New Zealand Companies Office as a Limited Company. Registration of a business name ensures that the name cannot be used by any other business. Registration is also a legal prerequisite when starting up a business in New Zealand. I also had to apply for an IRD number with the Department of Inland Revenue.

Name and logo

My business name, Creative Connections Arts Therapy, speaks clearly of the fact that I offer arts therapy services. I wanted my logo to represent something essential about my business and my therapeutic approach. My logo is simple, and includes my business name, as well as the words 'arts psychotherapy' and 'arts in the workplace' so that clients are able to gain an immediate understanding of what my business offers. The image is a playful combination of the letter A and a symbol, which is both a hand, and a tree with colourful leaves. (The hand makes reference to the fact that hands are used for making art, the tree is an allusion to my interest in eco-art therapy, and the brightly coloured leaves represent the potential colour and diversity of creative output.)

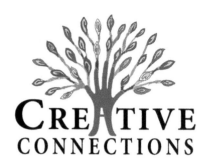

A logo is a great way to establish a brand identity, and I take every opportunity to increase the visibility of my logo on my business cards, my website, my business Facebook page, printed advertising, on invoices and receipts, and in all business-related email communication. There are advantages to ensuring that a business logo is visible on all marketing and communication, as it creates the impression that the business is professional, reputable and established.

In order to come up with a name and logo that worked, I found it very valuable to work with a symbol journal and, through this fluid and creative process, arrive at an image that encapsulated the essence of what I offer. A guided activity to creating a logo by using a symbol journal can be found at the end of this chapter.

Administration and finances

Income tax

As I am a little intimidated by the intricacies of income tax, I employ the services of an affordable and reliable accountant, who has recommended that I keep my personal and business bank accounts separate, and that business-related income is paid into that account only. I keep records of all business costs, such as computer-related expenses, web hosting fees, art materials and venue hire. Much of my work is done from home, and I am therefore able to claim a proportion of the interest paid on the mortgage, home and contents insurance, rates, power, mobile phone and internet fees. As my practice also involves a fair amount of travelling, I can claim a portion of my transport-related expenses.

Professional indemnity

I have selected to take out professional indemnity insurance. This would protect me from the financial liability if a client were to injure themselves while in my care. It would cover defence costs which could be incurred from a client complaint, or if allegations arose from a breakdown of a client relationship.

Contracts

When contracted by an organisation or business to facilitate an arts event, series of arts therapy sessions, or a one-off session, I request that we sign a formal contract. Larger organisations often have standard contracts for their contractors, but for those who do not I provide a contract which outlines my responsibilities as facilitator, as well as the logistical and financial responsibilities of the organisation contracting me. See Appendix 1 for an example of my standard contract.

I provide individual clients with a disclosure statement which outlines my credentials as an arts therapist, my therapeutic approach, and their rights as a client. This statement also provides an introduction to the therapeutic process, and gives some insight into what clients can expect from the therapeutic process, as well as an indication of my fee, and the bank details of the account into which payment should be made. I indicate that the fee is negotiable, and that there is a sliding scale for those in financial need. Welfare beneficiaries are advised how to go about applying to Work and Income New Zealand for a subsidy which covers a significant portion of the fee. I clarify that payment is due, in full, on the day of each session, and that receipts are sent out on a monthly basis. See Appendix 2 for a copy of my disclosure statement.

Invoices and receipts

I have found it useful to have templates for administrative documents, such as contracts, invoices and receipts, filed in a designated folder on my computer. I also keep soft and hard copies of all contracts, invoices and receipts.

Marketing

Social media

Online marketing via my website is proving to be an effective way for clients to access information about my business, and to contact me. In order to direct traffic to my website, and to reach out to new audiences, I have Facebook and Pinterest pages for my business. My Facebook business page, in particular, has provided me with a highly interactive platform for communication and marketing, and many of my clients have been introduced to my website and practice through this. Sharing news relating to group arts therapy sessions, arts events, as well as articles, links and images to my Facebook business page ensures that my business name, my logo, and my engagement with research and articles on arts therapy remain visible to the page followers. Their 'likes', shares and comments show up on their newsfeeds and introduce the page to their friends and followers. In order to keep my page interesting and informative, I endeavour to share a wide range of arts therapy and mental health related articles, as well as images and appropriate memes.

Creating a website

I chose to build my own website, using a web-building tool. This process has shown me that establishing an online identity is a work in progress, which involves many struggles, frustrations and some deadends. After limping through the early stages, and gaining an understanding of the technicalities involved, it became an easier and more fluid process. There are many do-it-yourself website builders, and it is well worth shopping around for a suitable web-building tool.

One of the first issues that I had to resolve related to my professional identity. Initially, I was unsure whether to present myself as an experienced and academically trained fine artist, who is also an arts therapist, or as an arts therapist who is open to the range and diversity of creative expression that my clients might bring to therapy. Reflecting on the emotional tug-of-war provoked by this professional identity crisis brought me to the realisation that there were deeper personal processes requiring consideration. It was with a great sense of relief that I decided to separate my identity as an arts therapist from my identity as an artist, and I now have two completely separate websites, one which serves as a platform for my arts therapy practice, and another to represent my fine art. The decision was motivated by my understanding that my website should reflect my client-centred approach, and serve as an introduction to the therapeutic service I provide, which is a safe space for my clients to explore and express their processes.

An important factor to consider when creating a website is the intended target market, as it is a good idea to gain an understanding of who will be accessing the information provided. I identify my potential target markets as residents of Auckland and the surrounding areas who wish to improve their wellbeing, or recover from mental health problems, by accessing arts therapy for themselves, or for their family members. Additional target markets are community, educational and corporate organisations who may benefit from arts in the workplace events. As so many members of the public are as yet unfamiliar with the benefits of arts therapy, I believe that it is important for my website to provide potential clients with an introduction to arts therapy, and to give answers to common questions which might be asked by clients, or parents who are considering arts therapy as a potential therapeutic option.

For the purpose of clarity, the homepage of my website provides a brief introduction to my business, to me, my qualifications, and the three services I provide, namely individual arts psychotherapy, group arts psychotherapy, and arts in the workplace events. More detailed information on these services is provided in separate pages, which are accessed via links from the homepage, or by clicking on the navigation bar. The 'about' page provides an introduction to my therapeutic approach. An 'information' page explains what clients can expect with regard to confidentiality, fees and boundaries, as well as a section which details their rights as a client. The 'contact' page enables clients to make email contact. It includes a Google Maps link to the address of my consulting rooms, and my mobile telephone number. As my business is not a crisis response service, I also include a section on this page which provides links and contact numbers to local emergency crisis services.

The 'client feedback' page contains examples of testimonials. Due to the confidential nature of the therapeutic relationship, feedback from clients in arts psychotherapy is always anonymous and can only be published if written feedback is volunteered, and if clients provide signed permission for its publication. Participants attending workshops, or arts in the workplace events, are invited to give written feedback on purpose-made feedback forms. These forms explain that participant responses may be used to advertise my business. (See Appendix 3 for a copy of my events feedback form.) The 'news' page links to the Facebook page of my business and is updated regularly as articles, images or updates are posted to my business Facebook page.

Printed media

In my experience, maintaining a visible presence in the community is important, and I regularly provide community centres, pharmacies and libraries with new and visually engaging posters for their notice boards. Brochures are another great way of making information on my business accessible to the public, and I make sure that these are displayed in appropriate places, like the brochure boards at local community centres. It is good practice to make use of all networking opportunities, and arts events and group arts therapy sessions for organisations provide suitable opportunities to hand out information flyers and business cards.

Developing an 'arts in the workplace' consultancy

The arts in the workplace events are aimed at enhancing group and individual motivation, goal-setting, and group and individual self-confidence by providing concrete, tangible, visible and experiential evidence of problem-solving, by demonstrating how mistakes can be transformed into creative learning opportunities. My aim is to give participants first-hand experience of how 'mistakes' can be transformed into creative learning opportunities when making art.

Workplace environments can be hierarchical, and often result in employees feeling stressed, exhausted, unappreciated and unmotivated. The arts therapy directives I use are adapted to suit workplace environments, and aim at enhancing motivation and mutual respect, and on strengthening corporate and team identity, while enhancing individual mental health and providing participants with a stronger sense of their own creative and personal potential. These events are geared to provide safe, contained opportunities for equalised participation, where hierarchies are temporarily and playfully suspended. The arts therapy processes utilised are non-threatening, and create potentially enjoyable ways to demonstrate how change is navigated, obstacles overcome, crossroads negotiated, helpful detours discovered, and goals set and reached.

Depending on what is required, sessions either begin with games aimed at encouraging a playful and informal mood, or with an exercise focused on breathing and mindfulness to enhance relaxation. Play, mindfulness and relaxation enable participants to be emotionally and physically present, and open to engagement with the therapeutic creative processes. The art experientials include group mandalas, large group paintings, woven life-lines, group puzzle paintings (where individuals work on their own images and then collaborate to fit them together to form a whole), group collages, as well as a range of directives focused on enhancing individual self-awareness, self-reflection and personal development. Participants in these sessions report enhanced wellbeing, self-confidence and self-awareness.

Market research

When first investigating the viability of the business, and opportunities available in this area, I looked at whether a potential market for arts therapy in workplaces could be established, and if there were other Auckland-based arts therapists who provided similar services. My online research focused on workplace attitudes towards employee health in New Zealand. My findings suggested that some organisations are aware that a positive focus on the mental health of their employees can potentially enhance productivity and wellbeing. This cursory investigation revealed that there was an acknowledgement of employee performance being negatively impacted by stress and other work-related pressures. The search also indicated that many companies provide employees with the means to reduce or address mental and physical health issues through the introduction of employer-assisted programmes which include healthcare training, psycho-education and counselling services, aimed at enhancing wellbeing. Employer-assisted programmes typically aim to provide support and referral for employees dealing with substance abuse, occupational stress, emotional and physical burnout, emotional distress, major life events, health problems, financial or legal problems, or work-related issues. Many of the large organisations and companies also provide medical insurance, which covers some psychotherapy, for their employees (EAP Services 2016).

In order to get a better understanding of how other arts therapists approach this environment, I conducted internet searches, focusing on terms like 'corporate arts therapy', 'arts therapy employee wellness', 'corporate group therapy', 'arts in the workplace' and 'employer-assisted arts therapy'. These searches revealed that there are a small number of arts therapists engaged in corporate practice in the UK, USA, South Africa and Australia, but that there are no other arts therapists promoting their practice to the workplace environment, or who have published articles relating to this field, in Auckland or New Zealand.

Arts therapists who provide services to workplaces, and who promote their practice online, emphasise the many potential benefits that arts therapy can have for that population. Their websites suggest that the psychological training of arts therapists enhances their insight into group dynamics, as well as an understanding of the way in which art can transcend verbal language. Other benefits cited include the fact that arts therapists are able to direct the creative process in order to yield meaningful and productive growth in their clients, and that the creative processes utilised by arts therapists provide fun, informal, innovative and interactive ways to release stress, facilitate creativity and innovative thinking, and improve team motivation, communication and morale, thereby improving workplace productivity (Arts in Health & Care 2003).

To gain practice in running arts in the workplace groups, I volunteered to facilitate arts therapy events for the management and staff of organisations where I completed clinical placements. Familiar people and organisational environments provided a great way to hone my skills in doing group work. Participants were invited to give written feedback, and informed that their feedback might be used to promote my arts therapy practice.

Marketing creative events to workplaces and organisations

The most effective way to establish a client base in this area is to be open to networking opportunities. I take every opportunity to give talks or demonstrations at schools (see Appendix 4 for an example of the covering letter I send to schools), present research papers at conferences, and facilitate arts therapy events for organisations. This ensures that I reach people, and groups, who may not otherwise have heard of arts therapy, or my business. Some of my most lucrative and successful contracts have been accessed in this manner, and I am endeavouring to build a reputation as a proactive group facilitator and clear communicator, by ensuring that my group sessions and workplace events are well organised, fun and meaningful experiences for everyone involved.

For many of my clients, the first introduction to my business is through my website. To ensure that potential corporate clients can access it, I include terms such as 'corporate arts therapy', 'employee wellness', 'corporate events' and 'arts in the workplace' in the SEOs (search engine optimisers) of my website (www. creativeconnectionsarttherapy.co.nz). The Arts in the Workplace page provides information on the service, and gives answers to some of the questions which new clients may have, by explaining that events aim at: enhancing communication skills and creative thinking; reducing work-related stress and the resulting mental and physical health problems; building team identity; and encouraging happiness, enthusiasm and wellbeing in the workplace. I clarify that events are creative, fun, versatile, non-threatening and enjoyable ways to navigate change, overcome obstacles, negotiate crossroads, discover new pathways, and set and reach goals. I explain that I utilise effective, evidence-based approaches, geared to: strengthening employee skills in critical areas such as communication, collaboration, conflict resolution, change management, intercultural communication and presentation; opening up possibilities for new models of team interaction; enhancing individual and team performance, productivity and workplace identity; improving employee mental health and wellbeing; accessing innate creativity and playfulness; and fostering creative thinking.

I have had some success from contacting organisations directly by sending an introductory email, followed by a phone call directly to an appropriate contact person. It is useful to establish the name and title, or position of the contact person. This can be done by doing online research, or by making telephone enquiries (see Appendix 5 for an example of my covering letter to corporate clients).

Case studies

- A successful facilitation of an arts therapy event at a corporate wellness retreat, organised by the business and law faculty of a local university, has led to further invitations to work with similar groups. The importance of networking and being open to business opportunities cannot be overemphasised, and events like these provide an ideal space to establish new connections. Brochures, business cards and feedback forms are made available to all participants, and complimentary art material packs clearly display my logo and business details.

- When approached by an organisation or group with specific needs with which I may be unfamiliar, I engage in research to find out more about their requirements. For example, after being approached to run arts therapy sessions for an organisation catering to people with aphasia, I made sure that I researched their specific requirements in order to gain an understanding of the needs of this population. The sessions were very popular, and the group members expressed great satisfaction, an enhanced sense of connection and communication skills, and feelings of wellbeing as a result. The success of this group has resulted in me being invited back to run another series of sessions for them, as well as invitations to facilitate ongoing groups for organisations who cater to people who have had strokes, and also groups with brain injury. After experiencing the benefits of arts therapy some group members have chosen to engage in individual therapy. I am in the habit of always carrying business cards with me, and I also make sure that I have brochures handy for those who request more detailed information.

- Advertising and facilitating an arts therapy group catering to immigrants has resulted in being invited to have an eco-arts therapy session with young immigrants filmed for a television programme, focusing on immigrant and refugee communities in New Zealand. Appearing on television is a great form of advertising for my business, and also serves to enhance the visibility of arts therapy to the wider community.

Conclusion

Starting out in private practice is proving to be an exciting and rewarding process. In the short term, I plan to continue building my client base, and as client numbers increase, I hope to be able to invite other local arts therapists to join my practice. In order to make my business appealing to future markets, I am aiming to enhance my online presence by blogging, as well as producing short YouTube films. A long-term goal is to establish a permanent arts therapy studio, which would include a well-equipped arts studio for groups, as well as cosy and inviting smaller spaces for individual arts therapy sessions.

Go and do it!

Exercise 1: The miracle question

This exercise is an adaptation of the solutions-focused therapy directive, the Miracle Question (de Shazer 1988). It is a useful way to begin to establish an idea of an ideal work and life scenario, and to find clarification with regard to goals, hopes and requirements. It is a way to focus attention on our greatest hopes, desires and aspirations, and to visualise an ideal life, without having to worry about the details of how to achieve it.

While sitting or lying down comfortably, close your eyes and relax. Breathe out and in with mindful awareness. When you feel completely relaxed, imagine that a miracle has taken place overnight, and all obstacles to you achieving all of your goals have vanished. Imagine yourself waking up in the most ideal and perfect place, all your hopes and dreams fulfilled. Look around and notice your environment. What do you see? Where are you? Who is with you?

Imagine yourself preparing for your day. What do you wear? Where do you work? Who do you work with? What do you do at work? Imagine how you spend your perfect working day. Notice all the details of your working environment.

Imagine that your working day is over. How do you feel? How do you spend the rest of your day? Pay close attention to all that you have imagined, and form pictures of what you have seen in your imagination. Notice what stands out for you. Imagine yourself making drawings, or taking photos of what you have seen. When you are ready, open your eyes, and make a picture of some of your most prominent memories from your visualisation.

Here are some suggestions on what to notice, and some questions you may wish to ask yourself when looking at your picture:

- Notice the important themes in your picture.

- What stands out for you?

- What surprises you?

- Are there elements, people or skills which already exist in your life?

- Are there any elements that are attainable in the short term?

- What can you do to set about reaching your short-term goals?

- Are there any elements that could be achieved in the long term, with perseverance and focus?

- What can you set in motion now in order to begin to achieve your long-term goals?

- How do you feel when you think of achieving your short-term and long-term goals?

Exercise 2: Find your logo: a symbol journal process

1. Choose a symbol that has meaning for you. It can be from anywhere, as long as it speaks to you.

2. Research your symbol by finding out what meanings ancient cultures or religions have associated with it. Find out if

there are any songs, stories, poems or films about it. Does it feature prominently in the work of a particular artist, or in popular culture?

3. Paste, draw and write these images and stories in your journal.

4. Once you have completed your research, draw your symbol in the centre of a page, and create a mind map of associations that relate to your symbol. Follow the different directions of the mind map to see where they lead. Try not to censor your thoughts, and fill the page with free associations.

5. Deconstruct your symbol. What is it made of? How is it made? How is it used? Where can it be found?

6. Consider the opposite aspect of your symbol, and translate this creatively by making an artwork in your journal.

7. Create a mind map of the shadow of your symbol in your journal. Include words associated with the shadow aspect of your symbol. Consider what is positive about the elements of the shadow. Think about the message that you can give yourself from your symbol's shadow.

8. Give your symbol a voice by writing a letter to it. Write a return letter to you, from your symbol.

9. Take the name of your symbol and use it in a sentence.

10. Consider what your symbol would look like if it was very large, or very small. Translate this creatively by making an artwork in your journal.

11. Consider how it would feature in a myth or fairytale, or what it would be like as a historical character. Translate this creatively by making an artwork in your journal.

12. Consider what it would look like if it were a body part, a quality in a relationship, an animal, or an object in nature. Translate this creatively by making an artwork in your journal.

13. Associate feelings you have with your symbol, and think about how these relate to qualities in yourself.

14. Explore your professional needs, values and life direction through the use of your symbol. Write down three general associations or attributes attached to these concepts, and then write them as 'I' statements.

15. Reflect on what you have learnt about yourself and your professional aspirations while undertaking these activities. In particular, what wisdom did the symbol share with you?

16. Using your symbol, and all that you have gathered from this process, create a logo that represents you, your art, and your professional approach.

References

Arts in Health & Care (2003, 26 June). Corporate art therapy. Retrieved from http://arttherapy.wordpress.com/2003/06/26/corporate-art-therapy on 30 November 2016.

de Shazer, S. (1988). *Clues: Investigating Solutions in Brief Therapy*. New York: W.W. Norton.

EAP Services (2016). Employee Assistance Programmes. Retrieved from www.eapservices.co.nz/employee-assistance-programes on 30 November 2016.

Appendices

Contract for arts in the workplace events/sessions for organisations

[Logo here]

[Name of Business]

Contract for the Provision of Arts Event/ Group Arts Therapy Session(s)

Between [name of business] .... and ....

This contract commences on [date] ....

Nature of Services

1. Arts in the workplace event/s, group arts therapy session(s)

2. This/these events will take place on [details of time, date] ......
....

3. At [venue] ....

Costs

1. The cost of venue hire will be covered by ....

2. The cost of art materials will be covered by ....

3. The cost of transport will be covered by ....

Responsibilities

1. [Name of business] .... agrees to provide .... with [number of events/sessions] .... arts in the workplace event/s, group arts therapy session/s, on/from [date/s] ....

Fees

1. The fee for the service will be ..../event/series of session(s) (including GST).

2. This fee includes/does not include art materials.

3. This fee includes/does not include transport.

Payment Terms

1. A deposit of 50% of total costs (fees, art material costs and transport costs) shall be paid within 24 hours of the signing of this contract.

2. The remaining 50% shall be paid within 24 hours of the service being delivered.

3. Fees shall be deposited into [bank account name] ....

   Bank account number ....

Terms

1. This contract shall commence on [date] .... to [date] .... unless it is terminated in one of the following ways:

   a) The parties mutually agreeing to terminate the agreement at an earlier date.

   b) One (1) month's written notice of termination by either party.

Acceptance of Terms and Conditions

I declare that I have read, and that I understand the terms of this contract, and that I fully accept them.

Signed: .... *Dated* ....

Signed: .... *Dated* ....

Name ....

Position ....

APPENDIX 2

Disclosure statement

[Logo here]

Welcome to my arts therapy practice. This disclosure statement outlines my credentials as an arts therapist, my therapeutic approach, and your rights as a client.

This statement also provides an introduction to the therapeutic process, and gives some insight into what you can expect from therapy.

If you have any questions about the content of this statement or about any aspect of your work with me, please don't hesitate to ask.

My qualifications

....

....

....

Professional affiliations

I am registered as an arts therapist with ....

My registration number is ....

Approach

As an arts therapist, I work within a person-centred, strengths-based, holistic framework. I hold the central hypothesis that everyone has an innate potential for personal awareness, psychological growth and the ability to express themselves creatively.

I provide individual and group arts as therapy, and arts psychotherapy services to clients across the life span. I use visual arts, and other expressive modalities, such as movement and play, as a way to help my clients explore and work through their problems. The process of engaging in arts therapy can entail the creation of visual art work, and other forms of creative expression.

I integrate approaches and techniques from various therapies and theories, such as attachment theory, clay therapy, cognitive behavioural therapy (CBT), dialectical behaviour therapy (DBT), eco-art therapy, expressive arts therapy, motivational interviewing, mindfulness, narrative psychology, positive psychology, psychodynamic arts psychotherapy, and solution-focused therapy.

What you can expect

I will be working alongside you in order to gain a deeper understanding of the issues which bring you to therapy. We will work together to cultivate skills and resources, provide insight into, and expand views of situations which you may be facing.

I aim to help you to find ways to live your life more effectively and creatively. We will explore your experiences, relationships, images and dreams in order to work towards recovery and to achieve your goals.

My role is to provide you with a non-judgemental space to express yourself creatively and verbally. I will provide you with feedback and guidance, but acknowledge that you are the expert on your life.

For parents and primary caregivers

If your child or adolescent is in therapy with me, I will endeavour to work with you and your child in order to provide insight into their problems. My aim is to help you to implement compassionate, creative strategies to support them in their development and recovery. I will aim to enable your child or adolescent to express their emotions, to have their emotions acknowledged, to heal from trauma and to interact positively in their home, school and social environments.

Risks and benefits

Arts therapy can sometimes feel nonlinear and unpredictable, but it can be one of the best ways to heal emotional wounds and to live life in more authentic and meaningful ways. Arts therapy can have benefits and risks.

The process often involves discussing unpleasant aspects of your life; you may experience uncomfortable feelings like sadness, guilt, anger, frustration, loneliness and helplessness. These feelings are usually temporary, and will generally diminish in time.

There are many benefits for those who go through this process. Arts therapy often leads to improved relationships, solutions to specific problems, and a significant reduction in feelings of distress. It can also enhance resilience, provide you with a better understanding of yourself, and lead to better parenting skills and communication skills.

The time it will take

The amount of time it will take to address the issues you bring to therapy will depend on your goals, the areas of concern, and the problems you choose to address. Some issues can be addressed in a few sessions, while others may take longer to resolve.

If you have chosen to focus on one issue, and find that the therapy has helped you to find resolution, you may decide to stop. You may want to explore deeper and more longstanding issues, which means that you may decide to spend more time in therapy.

You may wish to have weekly or fortnightly sessions, or you may find it comforting to establish a regular routine for your sessions. You are entitled to ask questions about the process, or to end the arts therapy process at any time.

Please bear in mind that it is most beneficial for the ending of therapy to be co-created. A planned ending will provide you with the opportunity to experience transitions or closure in a new and potentially more positive way.

Your rights

At your request, you have the right to receive information from me about the methods of therapy and the approaches used. You are also entitled to ask about the duration of your therapy, but should understand that this can often not be predetermined.

You are entitled to seek a second opinion from another therapist, or to terminate treatment at any time.

Your creative expressions

You are entitled to keep the creative expressions you make while in therapy. If you wish me to keep them for you, I will be happy to do so. You may take your creative work away with you when you decide to terminate therapy, or you may choose not to.

All your creative expressions will be treated with respect, be kept in a safe place, and will remain confidential.

Confidentiality

Our therapeutic work is confidential. That means that I will make every effort to keep private what you choose to share with me. Of course, you may choose to discuss your therapy with trusted others.

There are some limits to confidentiality. If I think that you or others are at risk of harm, I may need to speak with someone else (such as your GP). In this situation, I will always discuss my concerns with you first and inform you of any communication I may need to have to ensure your own, or other people's safety.

In some circumstances courts can take legal action to demand access to clinical notes. This only happens on rare occasions. I have confidential clinical supervision where I discuss my work with a colleague to ensure the high standard of my practice.

As a professional counsellor, information provided during the course of therapy is confidential except for situations described above.

Boundaries

If I meet, or see you outside of our session, I will only acknowledge or greet you if you initiate that. I do not initiate contact with clients in public spaces, or communicate through social networking sites. This is to protect your confidentially.

These boundaries continue even after counselling is terminated. This is an ethical obligation that benefits you by allowing me to serve as a therapist rather than a friend. Occasionally I may share some of my personal experiences in sessions, when it may be beneficial, but the focus will be on your experiences.

Feedback

I aim to provide you with a respectful and helpful arts therapy service. Please feel free to give any feedback about your experience of the way I work with you. Both criticism and praise are welcome, and both help me to provide a better, more tailored service for you. If you remain unsatisfied or wish to make a formal complaint this can be done via [name of professional affiliation] ....

Professional fee

My standard fee is .... per hour.

I will provide a negotiated sliding scale for those in financial need. Beneficiaries can apply to .... for a subsidy to cover the cost of their arts psychotherapy sessions.

Payment is due in full at the end of each session. I will provide you with a receipt for your session after payment is made.

If you choose to pay by direct bank deposit, you may do so. Please make your payment into the following account:

Account name: ....

Account number: ....

Cancellations

The time of your scheduled appointment is reserved for you. If you need to cancel or reschedule your appointment, please do so at least 24 hours in advance. It is my policy to charge for cancellations received with less than 24 hours' notice. No charge will be made for cancellations made with this notice.

Cancellations made on the day of the appointment with a minimum of four hours' notice may be charged at a rate of ....

Sessions cancelled or not attended with no notice given, or without 24 hours' notice, may be charged at the full rate.

Contact information

I can be reached on my mobile phone or by email.

My phone number is ....

My email address is ....

I am often not immediately available by phone. I do check my messages and emails regularly, and I will make every effort to return your call on the same day with the exception of Sundays and holidays.

If you are unable to reach me, and feel that you can't wait for me to return your call, you can call [number of emergency services] .... or contact your doctor. Other emergency services are listed on the contacts page of my website: ....

I have read the preceding information and understand my rights as a client. I have received an identical copy for my records.

....

Client signature   Date

....

Therapist signature   Date

APPENDIX 3

Creative events feedback form

[Logo here]

Please provide feedback. I value your opinion, and would appreciate knowing where I can improve. The feedback you provide may be included in marketing for [name of business] ....
.... arts events.

Please evaluate each statement according to the following scale:

1: Strongly agree 2: Agree 3: Neutral 4: Disagree 5: Strongly disagree

---

The facilitator

.... Was supportive

.... Was well prepared

.... Was engaging and interesting

.... Encouraged participation

The session

.... Helped me to express myself creatively

.... Helped me to relax, and enjoy the creative process

.... Provided useful/helpful ideas

.... Increased my understanding of how creativity can enhance my wellbeing

.... I would enjoy more opportunities like this to experience creative events

The art materials

.... Were appealing

.... Inspired me to explore my creativity

If you would like to be contacted by [name of business] ....
.... to discuss the possibility of arranging an arts
event for your workplace, please provide your name and contact details.

Name ....

Business/organisation name ....

Email address ....

Phone ....

Additional comments

....
....
....
....
....
....
....
....
....
....
....
....
....
....
....

APPENDIX 4

Example of an introductory email to schools

[Name of contact person (usually the principal, or school counsellor)]

[Title]

[School name]

Dear [contact person]

A free arts therapy demonstration for the parents and teachers of [name of school]

Many of us find it easier to communicate our emotions and experiences visually, rather than verbally. Art can be an effective tool for self-expression and communication. As a qualified and registered arts therapist, I am trained to understand visual communication, and to provide appropriate support, when it is needed.

I would like to offer the parents and teachers of [name of school] a free, 60-minute demonstration of how arts therapy can provide insight into personal processes and enhance wellbeing.

I am available to facilitate the demonstration when it is most suitable for the school, the teachers and the parents. I am offering this demonstration at no cost, but would like to request that a suitable venue, for example a classroom or meeting room, be made available. I am also happy to cover the cost of the art materials used, but request that those who are interested RSVP for planning purposes.

If you would like to find out more about arts therapy, and how it can work, please visit my website at [website address].

I look forward to your response, and will be happy to talk with you over the phone, or meet with you to discuss this further.

Yours sincerely

[Name]
[Qualification]
[Registration details]
[Business name]

APPENDIX 5

Example of an introductory email to workplaces or organisations

[Business name]
[Business address]
[Addressee (the name of the HR manager, or appropriate contact person)]

Dear [Name]

Arts in the Workplace events

Did you know that introducing creativity in to the workplace is a well-recognised and effective way to enhance employee performance? The creative workplace events I provide use evidence-based, fun, non-threatening and versatile methods to:

- resolve workplace conflict
- enhance communication skills and encourage creative thinking
- reduce work-related stress and the resulting mental and physical health problems
- build team identity
- encourage happiness, enthusiasm and wellbeing in the workplace
- navigate change, overcome obstacles and negotiate crossroads
- discover new pathways, and set and reach goals.

As a qualified, registered arts therapist I offer experience in the facilitation of creative workplace events, as well as unique insight into personal and team dynamics and processes. I have a broad range of service offerings that I can tailor to the needs and requirements of your organisation. If you would like to find out more about [business name], please visit [website address].

I look forward to following up with you by phone in the near future in order to arrange a meeting with you.

Yours sincerely

[Name]
[Qualification]
[Registration details]
[Business name]

CHAPTER 9

Case Study: Managing Business Growth from the Bottom Up
Turning Your Small and Niche Passion into a Business

Vicky Abad

Introduction

Many businesses begin with a clear business plan that grows from an idea that someone is very passionate about; they have a vision of where they want to go and implement a strategy to get there. This kind of business planning rings true to the saying 'Start the way you wish to continue.' My business started with a passion, but not a plan. It grew from the heart, not the head. This has led to many wonderful and life-enriching moments as well as many business challenges. This chapter provides an account of how Boppin' Babies came to be, and examines how this small business grew in order to provide an excellent customer experience and a family-friendly work environment, and meet the ever-changing market forces of the 21st-century economy. I hope that you find it interesting and useful in your own personal business journeys.

Transitions in life, transitions in work

In 2006 my life took a new direction that marked a significant change in my working life. I had been working as a registered music therapist for over 10 years, starting out as a sole proprietor predominately in aged care facilities. I believe these early years of navigating contracts, pay rates, insurance and networking – from the Director of Nursing and the Registered Nurse on duty through to the other allied health teams, the office staff who paid my invoices and the kitchen staff who served hot chocolates during our evening relaxation and music appreciation group – placed me in good stead to revisit the self-employment model many years later. After this period of self-employment I took an employed position at a children's hospital before moving into the community sector and working closely with government to set up a large music therapy early-intervention service for parents and children. All of this changed in 2006 when I took leave to have my first child.

Motherhood

When my daughter was born I moved from being the therapist who worked with mothers to being the mother. Becoming a mother impacted heavily on the way I worked with other mothers and clients in general. I had spent the past six years building an early-intervention programme that focused on creating a welcoming, safe and therapeutic experience that allowed parents (predominately mothers) to bond with their infants and learn about the importance of positive parenting, and highlighting ways that music supported early childhood development. Now I was the mother. The importance of all of this seemed even more paramount. It also seemed more pertinent to all parents. As a therapist, I had worked with clients with complex needs. Now, as a mother myself, I moved in mother circles and observed that all mothers, from all walks of life, were after information on how to be good in this new mothering role. There were plenty of parents, including myself, wanting information on parenting, including how to be attuned to their child's needs and be the very best parent that they could be.

As I moved in these new circles, I also observed that musical parenting was not always present in the dyadic relationships I observed. These kinds of interactions have been described by Malloch as 'communicative musicality' (Malloch & Trevarthen 2009). These parents were not 'at-risk' like my previous client group had been, and yet, here we were looking for ways to do our best. I knew that music was a powerful tool for parents if they were looking for ways to be attuned to their child. One week, I took my guitar to my mother's group and improvised to the mood of the group, playing a few children's songs for the babies and singing some lullabies. There was a lovely calmness as many babies went to sleep and mothers took a moment to relax and simply be. It was a beautiful moment. One mother said to me,

'What did you just do?' I explained I used the music to entrain the babies and changed the pace, timbre, and my voice, to put them to sleep. We had a chat about how the mums could do this at home. At the end of the group one of the mothers said to me, 'Wow! You should be charging us for this! That was sublime.' I began to think about how I could make this information and my skills available to families who were not able to access government-funded programmes.

At the same time that these thoughts entered my head, I had begun looking for a music programme to take my own child to. I wanted to be in the musical moment with her, as her mum, and share this special time together while she was still so little, yet I found the classes I went to did not support my child's innate musicality, or facilitate musical interactions between us like I knew music could do so beautifully. I found this frustrating and sad. At the time I wrote the following excerpt in my journal, and this has been used as part of my PhD reflections on what drove me to research why parents seek out music groups for their infants in the first place:

> Today as I sat on the floor, surrounded by other mothers and their babies, I felt a profound sense of sadness and disappointment that this music class, like the others we tried, was not what I was led to believe. The teacher did not sing in key. She used recorded music to engage and interact with babies that were too young to be prescribed to. There was a lack of personal attention that music so beautifully invites. There was no support for the musical interactions that I know music can inspire. I feel really disappointed because I have looked so forward to this for so long – a time in my life where I get to share my love of music with my love – my baby. I feel sad too for the other people in the room – maybe they don't know that this class was not all that it could be, or all that it promised? Do they know the potential power that music has to provide a moment in time for a mother and her child to simply 'be' – to take delight in each other, to share musical interactions, to smile and laugh and touch and share? I have provided this to others for years, now I would love to be able to share it with my own little one. Put simply, a musical place to bond and interact with my baby in a musical environment where we could be equal musical participants. But this would require a programme that understood early childhood development, the musical development of infants, the power of music to act as an agent for communication and attachment

between a mother and a child, a highly skilled musician, an informed group leader, and someone who could empower the mothers to take home the music learnt and use it with their babies in their everyday interactions... Maybe it should be me? But then who gets to be mum to my bub while I take the group? Are the other parents here for the same reason? To share a moment in time? To take delight? Or do they believe what the programme promised in regards to smarter children, or are they starting music education early thinking it will give their child a head start? What motivates these parents to bring their babies to a music programme, to dress them, pack them up, get them in the car, go into the music room – so much planning, so much doing... so much money...

After this music class, I remember driving home and singing to my baby while she fell asleep in the car. That afternoon we played and sang as we always did and it occurred to me that I was doing exactly what I wanted a music programme to do. I was being in the musical moment with her, using life and responsive music to interact, to love, to play, to learn together, and to simply be. So I started taking one music group a week that my daughter could attend. Instead of being her parent I once again was the facilitator but a beautiful thing happened instead – she came with her father and they shared this beautiful musical moment. It was a blessing and an honour to be able to provide this for my family and for the families that joined us.

Starting a business

Starting a business with a five-month-old baby was not in my plans. My priority was being a mother and supporting my infant child to grow, and to use music to do this, not to run a business. I had planned to return to work after maternity leave, but found that full-time employment did not work for as a parent. But that is another story. However, the need for an interactive parent–child music programme became obvious to me and I began to think about how I could meet this need in the community.

Many businesses start with a clear outline, its plan and objectives mapped out, its financial goals clearly articulated. I began with the idea that I could meet my child's needs with a music group, and from there, provide interactive parent–child music groups one small group at a time. I decided to start slowly and build only when there was time and space, as the music group was secondary to my parenting responsibilities at the time. Opportunity for growth came via word of mouth. As my daughter grew the business grew, one group to two, always slow, always balanced with her.

At this point in time I needed a business name. I reflected on what it was that I loved so much about the groups and how I could capture this in a name. I loved the parents and their babies interacting musically, bonding together, and I loved the way the babies bopped up and down to the music that first time they realised they could move their bodies in time with me – I loved that we could be entrained musically and share this amazing musical journey together. The name Boppin' Babies was born.

When my baby became a toddler I started one toddler group in addition to the baby groups. Toddlers' needs were very different so I kept using live music and the very flexible and child-led model that I had used with the babies, which allowed me to follow their lead and let them be with their parents in the musical moment. At this time many of my baby boppers were moving into childcare and parents asked if we could provide services in centres. I wasn't able to meet this need at the time, and will reflect on that later.

Then my baby became a pre-schooler, so I started a pre-school group with her. I noticed she was more inquisitive about how we were making music with our bodies and our voices and I also noticed how beautifully she had flourished musically. She was now ready to start learning about music in a more formalised way, so this was when I started introducing music education principles into the groups. When my daughter started school the business really took off. Now I had some time to respond to need and implement some programmes that had been on the waiting list for years.

Growing a business

During this period of business growth I responded to a number of issues that had been building up over time. These included:

- expanding the locations of our groups so that more families could access the programme in a wider variety of geographic locations

- starting a childcare programme that met the needs of families whose children moved into care

- providing free events for all to access.

Brisbane covers a large geographical space and is divided by a river. Many people were enquiring about attending Boppin' Babies but were not able or willing to drive across town to access services. The first business expansion we did was to offer more groups in different geographic locations around the city. There were advantages and disadvantages to doing this. The most obvious advantage was the fact we could now offer more services to more people in their local communities. This built local community capacity as much as it did our business, as parents would come together, form friendships, play in the local parks, buy coffees at the local coffee shops, and support each other in their parenting journeys. We could also offer more work to local music therapists, further building local community capacity. The challenges of this kind of expansion, though, are plenty – sourcing a decent community space to run a group at an affordable price is tricky to say the least. One disadvantage to this expansion model was moving away from a potential 'studio' space, where we could have purpose-built a music therapy and music early learning space specifically to fit the needs of children. This would have been geographically limiting though, so we went for accessing community space in multiple locations.

The second growth challenge was to adapt our programme to suit childcare settings where there were no parents present. This was achieved by adapting session plans to have a greater developmental focus and then collaborating with an independent organisation who was given licence to use the Boppin' Babies programme in childcare. This meant they managed the human resources of expansion, freeing up my time to develop the curriculum and recruit and train new staff.

The third growth challenge was finding ways to make what is essentially a user-pay programme accessible to most despite the costs involved. As a music therapist who came from a not-for-profit background, I wanted to find ways to provide free and equitable services to all families as well as providing a user-pay model to those looking for additional services. We achieved this by establishing partnerships with local governments and corporations to provide free music events for families in community spaces.

So as you can see here, Boppin' Babies has grown quite a bit from the original one group. This business model has evolved from a grass-roots level. Let's explore some of these moments of success and some of the challenges presented by growing a business organically.

Building a business from the bottom up

Boppin' Babies celebrates and supports the musical interactions between a parent and their child. At the time the business started, the only services that offered a similar experience were government-funded and available only to families deemed 'at-risk'. Other music programmes available for babies were more educational and less flexible in what they offered. I felt there were many parents looking for a different kind of programme and level of support who had no access to government-funded programmes. Thus I offered a user-pay system where parents could sign up and pay for a term and attend music with their child. The business grew out of a local need and expanded in response to this need over real time via locally aimed and driven grass-roots marketing.

Running a business requires a very different skill set to being a contractor or an employee. I had worked for myself previously, but there was one enormous difference in what I was now doing: working directly with paying clients. There was no government money coming in to subsidise or support my programme; I had to 'sell' a service to people and make my own way economically. As a self-employed music therapist working in aged care many years ago, the money that paid my invoices was provided by the government to the nursing home. While there was always a chance of losing the funding due to government cutbacks, the money was generally secure and I was paid each month. As an employee at the children's hospital and at Sing&Grow, a community-driven music therapy project, the government also paid my wages. My client was not the person who paid me. Now I sold directly to the consumer. And when you sell something you love dearly, it can feel personal when people don't want the service you offer. Before, as an employee, I viewed feedback through a professional lens. And while this should always be the case, it requires a great deal of discipline to keep your professional lens on when the business is something very personal to you. Thus, there are advantages and disadvantages of starting up a small business based on your passion, and growing this small business from the ground up. Here are some that are personal to my experience, that you may (or may not) find useful to reflect on as you start up your own business.

Advantages:

- Live in the moment! Love what you do.
- Realise and grow your dream and build your dream job within that.
- Be truly passionate about what you do.
- Fit work/business in with your lifestyle.
- Working in the business (not just on the business) means it is hands-on, so you don't lose sight of what people actually want.
- It is affordable.
- Organic growth – no funding upfront or loans to worry about (in my case).
- Niche business, unique set of skills/training/music therapy.
- Working closely with colleagues who are also your friends.
- Providing services to families who may also be your friends.

Disadvantages:

- No vision beyond the here and now (also a strength but not for a business).
- Risk of outgrowing your idea quickly if early planning did not scope out what the business might become:
  » outgrowing the space
  » outgrowing the name
  » outgrowing time/resources – scope to provide services.
- If your client group is also your friend group this can lead to awkward moments when managing a business, such as running accounts, or managing group dynamics.

- It is personal so it is hard to not take things personally:
  - » when friends move on to other businesses
  - » when people don't like your marketing/comments, etc.
- Being niche makes it hard to scale up.
- Employing colleagues in a small profession is fraught with danger.
- Training takes time and money – using registered music therapists (RMTs) can be expensive and hard to source as we are a small profession and people move on.

From the bottom to the top, challenges in between

Today, Boppin' Babies provides music early learning experiences and parent support to families with children aged from zero to four years. In addition to this, it provides ongoing music therapy and music education services for families beyond the first years of life through two sister companies. The business employs music therapists, music teachers, office administrators and communication and marketing specialists, as well as contracting the services of other therapists. Some days I reflect how it has grown from the bottom up to provide services to many thousands of children and families in both community and childcare settings. And I reflect on the amount of work I now provide to other music therapists and teachers and income to local businesses. I am also proud to generate an income that is independent of government funding so that I am supporting the community that I live in through tax generation.

What does it look like at the bottom?

At the bottom of this model, it looks fun! We make music all day with children and their parents in our music early learning groups or in our music therapy sessions. We teach music to children before and after school and we run free school holiday programmes! We conduct music therapy sessions in people's homes and at schools and community centres. My daughter once explained to a friend what I do by saying, 'She sings to babies and makes them happy, and she helps little children learn and grow with music.' It certainly is a fun and rewarding job.

What does it look like in the middle?

In the middle it is busy! We are busy planning sessions and writing plans behind the scenes, staying in touch with parents, booking people in for trials, following up enquiries, recording session notes, responding to requests for certain activities and events, meeting with people, planning for the next terms, meeting other businesses, setting up partnerships, planning our growth.

What does it look like at the top of the model?

At the top of the model, it looks amazing! It looks big! It looks overwhelming, and it can be lonely. This is where worlds can collide. Running a business and being a therapist require very different skill sets. I need to make a profit, I need to charge fees, I have staff to pay and a family to feed. Not all therapists are comfortable with the idea of making money, as opposed to taking money from a government-funded position. However, at the end of the day, it is a wage – I pay others, and I need to pay myself. This requires economic decisions to be made about how much I charge for services (what we offer) and pay for services (staff time and employment) and these are set in accordance with both government awards and market value. When you work in an industry as small as music therapy, you will likely employ colleagues and often friends, making some of these decisions difficult at best. One of the ways that I have managed this is to work with third parties that have licence to use the programme and therefore are responsible for employing colleagues. The other way I manage this is to have very clear contract of employment and protocols in place to manage HR.

Defining a business that has grown up

Boppin' Babies has grown up with my family. It has grown out of my experience as a music therapist and I identify as a music therapist when I work in the business. I don't, however, define it as a music therapy business. Rather, I define it as a music early learning programme (MELP). Currently there is no working definition of a MELP. Margaret Barrett, Professor of Music at the University of Queensland, and I have been working on devising one as part of our ongoing research work together. We define it as 'a program that has been designed by a qualified music teacher or registered music therapist with the intention of nurturing a love of music, supporting musical and extra-musical development in the child, and empowering the parent to use music in the home' (Abad & Barrett 2016, p.139).

The business growth from a music therapy perspective is clear when we review the two main beliefs that I have used to inform business practice. These are (1) that children are inherently musical, and (2) that parents are their children's first and most influential teachers. This first belief informs my practice in using music to support and enhance early childhood development by connecting with the musical child (Nordoff & Robbins 1977). The second influences the way the programme is offered, always with a parent present, and always within a model that empowers and supports parents to take music and use it back in their homes and in their everyday musical parenting practices. This feeds back to those earliest observations I reflected on when I first became a mother: I observed many parents looking for ways to connect with and be attuned to their babies, and professionally and personally I knew music could provide this.

Boppin' Babies supports child development through active music making, and knowledge of how music and development interact, overlap and work together. In particular, the programme aims to support sequential development through a focus on: multi-modal stimulation and sensory awareness and development in baby groups; social skills development, sensory integration and regulation in toddler groups; and pre-academic skills, emotional and social regulation and development, and motor skill coordination in pre-school groups, as well as the beginning of music awareness and education (Abad &

Barrett 2016). Boppin' Babies supports parents to use music in their everyday parenting by providing resources, ideas and mentoring on how to use musical songs, games and activities in the home (Abad & Barrett 2016).

Reflections on business growth and growing pains

Boppin' Babies began with my own parenting journey, and it began providing services for babies. The name reflects this very well. You now know that the business has grown and expanded and now provides services for toddlers, pre-schoolers, primary-aged children, adolescents and adults! We outgrew our own name! We outgrew venues and locations; we could not host enough groups with an average booking rate of 95 per cent and retention rates of 90 per cent per term. We outgrew the booking systems, record keeping systems, and we also outgrew staff requirements, having in fact outstripped local supply in the profession. When you grow a business from the ground up you sometimes don't see how big it is getting and the need for change creeps up on you! This section will reflect on some issues that crept up on me and the growing pains experienced as a result, and ways you can prepare yourself for this too.

What's in a name?

A business name is pivotal to the success of your business. Some people choose names that convey the expertise, value and uniqueness of the product or service they offer, while others will choose names that are broader, and allow for an association to be made and for growth to occur under the one umbrella. I chose a specific name that quite literally reflected the activity that we do – babies bop to music. This is useful for conveying the core business for the babies, but as I have outlined, the business now provides services to a larger market. This has led to the difficult decision of whether to rebrand the business to allow for greater growth with all populations, or create sister companies to work alongside the original and core business.

Ultimately, a good marketing strategy will allow you success with both, but here are some things for you to consider going forward:

- Choose a name that allows you to grow with it or into it.

- Choose a name that captures your unique business angle in a way that doesn't restrict you *or* stick to niche and let the name reflect your speciality.

- Decide if you want the words 'music' or 'therapy' in the name: these words can play to your advantage or hinder your growth.

Read Daniel Thomas' case study in Chapter 10 of this book for more reflections on this topic.

As Boppin' Babies grew from a baby to a toddler, pre-schooler and primary schooler itself, the question was to change or not to change the name. To change names meant there was a risk of losing market value as people might not transition with us to the new name. Our plan was to rename but not rebrand, in an effort to carry through with our successful branding model; however, in the end, for us, it made more sense to keep the name and expand with sister companies.

Managing a business

When I started this business it was small and manageable to run on my own. It was a 'small business', also known as a lifestyle business (see Chapter 10 by Daniel). That is – it suited and funded the lifestyle I wanted at the time. It grew bigger, and consequently new systems were required to manage data, attendance, staff employment, and many other things. A word of advice in this area: plan ahead. Look for systems that complement each other and help you avoid doubling up. Time is my currency. Systems that duplicate waste my time. For example, use an accounting system that also sends invoices and has a payroll; use a booking system that also allows you to establish a database and email system and feeds directly into a newsletter platform. Look for payment systems that allow clients to pay online *and* feed into your accounting systems. Some things for you to consider going forward:

- Check out Xero account managing systems.

- Look for a platform like PayPal that allows online payments.

- Look for calendars that can be shared, like the Google calendar app.

- Look for practice management software if you book a lot of therapy sessions.

Getting the word out there

When I started Boppin' Babies, business advertising was fairly basic for small businesses. Local marketing was key to many small businesses, often in the form of a self-produced brochure. People were really just starting to use websites to promote businesses. Social media did not really exist yet, especially not for business. Nowadays, social media plays a vital part in many small businesses and with my client base, mothers and parents, I would go so far as to say it is an essential part of marketing. This can be a great way to get the word out to local families. However, there are some very important things to be aware of when you set up your social media accounts:

- Know your audience well. Know what platform best suits your audience – Twitter, Instagram, Facebook, the list goes on and on. Remember time is a currency – managing all these platforms will take a *lot* of time.

- Know the rules of each platform and keep up to date – they change all the time.

- Pick one or two and do them really well.

- Know the rules of engagement for your profession. Some music therapy bodies and other allied health professional bodies have rules around testimonials. For example, in Australia, music therapist are not allowed to get or use these in their business practices, and this includes Facebook reviews.

- Know when to switch off: a ridiculously harder concept than it sounds when these platforms run 24/7 and the expectation is that you will be available to people quickly (Facebook even rates your time in responding to messages and this is publically available on your business page for clients to see).

Managing your time – a word on busy

If your small business is successful, chances are it will not stay small for long. Be prepared for being busy, but also be prepared to manage your busy so it doesn't manage you! Busy seems to be the new endemic of this century! It is hard to not be busy for the sake of being busy these days, with so many platforms to manage, so much data and information at hand to review all the time, and so many social media accounts to monitor! These days we are plugged in permanently, information is coming at us 24/7. What to do…

Busy has become such a phenomenon that Tony Crabbe wrote a book on it – *Busy: How to Thrive in a World of Too Much* (2014). In this book he defines busyness as 'that frenetic, always alert, multitasking that propels us through overburdened lives. It involves being always "on", glancing regularly at our phones and jumping from task to task. It is the juggling, cramming, and rushing that makes up so much of our daily existence. It is urgency, distraction and exhaustion' (Crabbe 2014, p.xi).

Busy is inevitable in the 21st century but it is not good for you or your business, and yet it is a very real part of running a small business. Here are a few of the hats I wear that make me sometimes feel overwhelmed with busy and busyness:

- manager of people
- office administrator
- Facebook guru (I'm joking. Facebook learner driver – it changes constantly)
- social media accounts manager
- marketing manager
- accounts manager
- human resource manager
- clinical manager
- supervisor
- researcher
- clinician – reading, planning, doing, reflecting, learning

- teacher

- mentor

- office cleaner.

Then add the rest of my life, things I don't want to take second place to business but sometimes unwittingly do:

- family – being a parent, wife, daughter, granddaughter, and so many other roles within the family

- extra-curricular activities for my child (sport, music, choir)

- running a household

- having my own friends and maintaining these relationships

- nurturing my own love of music

- exercising for fun and for health.

These lists could go on and on…the problem here is obvious to many: you start a small business to fit in with your family and then that small business takes over your family time and, if you allow it, your life! Add to this the very real fact that busy is bad for your health if ongoing stress is something you experience day in and day out. Stress is not all bad. It helps us to perform at peak and under pressure. But as John Medina describes is his book *Brain Rules* (2008), our brains and bodies are designed for short sharp assaults of stress hormones like adrenalin and more specifically cortisol, not long-term ongoing exposure. In fact, long-term exposure to stress hormones affects our immune system and even our ability to remember and learn new things (Medina 2008). This can't be good for you, your family, or your growing business. Crabbe (2014) lists a few things that busy is bad for and they include your business! The first victim of busyness is relationships, followed by happiness, career and business (Crabbe 2014). If you run a small business, make no mistake, there will be a *lot* to do, but as Crabbe says, 'busyness isn't essential. Yes there is a lot to do,' he tells us, 'but believing you're always busy because you have so much to do is both false and unhelpful. Busyness is a normal response to a world of too much, but it isn't the only response' (Crabbe 2014, p.xv).

If you fear you have succumbed to busy, and I can personally relate to that, then read Tony Crabbe's book and equip yourself with ways to master 'busy'. Ultimately, he believes that 'too much' is here to stay, so we need to change the way we do busy. In the meantime, here are some very simple steps I have adopted and some things for you to consider going forward:

- Turn off your social media accounts in the evening. Consider taking them and your email off your phone so that you have some physical separation from these. There are many advantages to quick and easy access when working for yourself, but sometimes you also need a clear break. If you keep them on the phone, practise self-discipline and don't check the accounts at night after a specified time.

- Set specific times to check your accounts throughout the day (outlined above) rather than having them open all the time while you are working. The constant pinging is distracting and if you are tempted to check them you will lose precious time re-focusing onto your current task.

- Set time boundaries with staff. State when you are available for meetings/emails and when you are not. Set 'no-go' times that are exclusive to family (such as the time before dinner or immediately after school) and explain to staff you won't be meeting, checking emails or taking calls during that time. Set time for staff that won't be interrupted by family.

- Have a schedule for administrative tasks as much as possible. Lock set tasks (accounts, enquiries, caseload revisions) onto set days at set times and try your hardest to stick to it.

- Have some time every week to work *on* your business not just *in* it. Being busy often means you get so caught up doing that you have no time for the planning and growing.

Being a leader

Starting your own business will be fun and rewarding. It will be hard work. You will be amazed at the things you didn't know you could do and at your success! The business may be like another child: it will please you and at other times really upset you. But you will love it all the same. I started a business in a new clinical area not commonly worked in by music therapists. I have pushed music therapy programmes into new clinical areas before and while this is exciting it can also be exhausting. If you are the same, you are a leader! Congratulations! This is a great thing, but being a leader means you have to have big shoulders. Many will let you push through to new areas, while often being quite critical, but then happily come up along behind you, on the path you have trod for them. This comes with the territory so there is no point being upset when it happens. In addition to setting the way, sometimes in the creative arts therapies you may also come across people who are not qualified in the field at all following along your path and using it to inform businesses or work of their own. Knowing this upfront will help you manage feelings that may arise about others 'copying' or following in your footsteps. Think of it as a form of flattery. I remind myself all the time that it is a great thing if more people are offering truly excellent services and enriching children's lives with access to music. If I don't believe them to be excellent, or they are not led by appropriately qualified staff, then I work even harder to set an even higher standard for people to aspire to.

Another term I hear used a lot for people like myself is 'pioneer'. Again, it is a great honour to be identified as one and I am very proud of the great programmes I have set up and the many jobs I have created. This role, however, dances precariously closely with the busy dance. There is a need to have clear boundaries so that while the pioneering work you do is of benefit to the profession, it is not to the detriment of your own family, health or business. You still need to feed your family and have a healthy work–life balance so you can service your clients and provide employment for yourself and your staff. Too much time pioneering may lead to not enough time for business. The building of a profession needs to be shared among many. Be a leader and a pioneer by all means, but encourage your colleagues to share the workload that is required to break new ground and gain recognition for your profession.

The end plan

When I started Boppin' Babies I had a niche view of what the business would be and who it would service. I set it up quite specifically for my young daughter and it grew from there. At that time, I didn't stop and think 'What is my end plan? Where will I go from here?' In hindsight, these kinds of questions would have been very helpful in planning for the growth. My colleague Daniel Thomas has taught me much in this area. Why? Because running a small business that becomes a larger business is hard work. There are no sick days, holidays are unfunded and some days it encroaches on family time and the very lifestyle you set it up to support. Boppin' Babies is now a family business run by more than just me. Building a business with replicable systems is different to running a small business. Knowing the end plan allows you to build, replicate, and provide greater scope and service. For the business to run without you at the epicentre you need to plan and systemise. This is where we are now (we being my family who run this business with me). It has been an amazing journey to date and one that we will continue with into the future. We learn as we go and this case study has aimed to help you learn and plan for your business growth, whether that growth is to maintain your small business as a niche service, to run it as a lifestyle business, or to expand and take over the world! Whatever it is you do, do it well, do it with passion, do it with love and be sure to remember to have fun along the way. You will be busy, you will be stressed, but ultimately you are the master of this universe and you can create it how you want.

Go and do it!

Exercise 1: What's in a name?

In Chapter 8, Elaine Matthews Venter asked you to go find your logo. Now I'm suggesting you reflect on your name if you have one, or find one if you don't.

- Close your eyes, visualise what it is you love about your business, about what you actually do – open them and write down three words that capture that vision or feeling.

- Can they be written into a name that will allow other people to visualise what you do without seeing your business in action?

Exercise 2: Manage your busy

- Choose three administrative tasks you find yourself doing daily, and schedule three set times a week to do these tasks in the one time frame. These should be tasks you don't have to do daily, but rather, tasks you do find you do daily and therefore eat into your time. An example of this would be to return phone calls at three set times a week rather than immediately after a session/meeting (if the call is not urgent).

- Schedule three time points to check your emails each day. Then close your emails down.

- Pick one hour a week to *read* about your professional area.

- Pick one hour a week and sanction it for *you* time, no work.

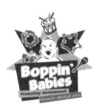

References

Abad, V. and Barrett, M. (2016). Families and Music Early Learning Programs – Boppin' Babies. In S. Jacobsen and G. Thompson (eds), *Models of Music Therapy with Families (pp.135–151)*. London: Jessica Kingsley.

Crabbe, T. (2014). *Busy: How to Thrive in a World of Too Much*. London: Piatkus.

Malloch, S. and Trevarthen, C. (2009). Musicality: Communicating the Vitality and Interests of Life. In S. Malloch and C. Trevarthen (eds), *Communicative Musicality: Exploring the Basis of Human Companionship (pp.513–530)*. Oxford: Oxford University Press.

Medina, J. (2008). *Brain Rules: 12 Principles for Surviving and Thriving at Work, Home and School*. Victoria: Scribe.

Nordoff, P. and Robbins, C. (1977). *Creative Music Therapy*. New York: John Day & Co. [Out of print]

CHAPTER 10

Case Study: Independence, Passion and Resilience
Learning to Think Big from the Start
Daniel Thomas

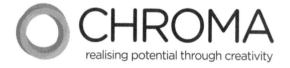

Introduction

Being successful is often a result of keeping going. My first business was a flop; the idea was great, the market was there, but I lacked any understanding of the finances – the primary school newspaper I created with a friend cost six pence to produce but we sold it for five. Thankfully, the 'Bank of Mum' stepped in and bailed us out. In our defence, we were only seven years old. The lessons from *The School Times* newspaper incident are useful for any new business, highlighting the importance of answering three key questions at the outset:

- Does it work?

- Will it sell?

- Will people pay for it?

Thinking therapeutically about why I have been either self-employed or an employer, with brief skirmishes into the world of employment, the impact of my parents' divorce, when I was aged eight, seems a key moment. As a result of the divorce, I needed to become more independent, developing a capacity to think for myself and go it alone. The situation also required resilience and any that I already had may have been enhanced. My other salient memory, which in hindsight seems linked to being entrepreneurial (or improvisational), occurred in the run-up to Christmas 1981 with Miss Wilson, my piano teacher. I had been asked to learn 'White Christmas' for the school panto, which I did, but I also embellished the sheet music version with passionate improvisational flourishes. Upon playing my version to Miss Wilson, she commented that although my version was 'all well and good' it wasn't what was written on the page. 'Yes I know!' I exclaimed in joy, but then stormed out in tears, ripping up the manuscript as I went (for maximum effect) as I realised that for Miss Wilson, playing correctly was more important than improvising and connecting with passion or joy.

Passion and resilience are two things we need in bucketloads to have a chance at being successful in business. To manage an arts therapy business, you need even greater amounts due to the non-mainstream nature of the services offered. This is slowly changing, but learning to embrace rejection – 'the No' – is a key step in the process. If self-employed therapists and therapist employers train themselves to hear 'the No' as an opportunity to look for 'the Next Yes', their passion and resilience form a series of creative and improvisational (or entrepreneurial) actions on a pathway to success. Sticking around long enough to allow success to happen and learning from the mistakes that will occur is the other part of the jigsaw.

Making an omelette, breaking an egg

My interest in running an arts therapy business started gradually and developed organically from 2005. Graduating in 2002 from the Welsh College of Music and Drama (WCMD), I took on a wide range of music therapy work in an attempt to find client groups I enjoyed working with, and to earn enough money to put food on my table. My mentality back then was to earn just enough to cover my rent, food and other normal monthly expenses. The reality of this meant I worked three days a week and had plenty of spare time; whilst often enjoyable, this sometimes led to isolation. Being independent, however, I was able to find, create and secure music therapy work that no one else was doing in my area. I set up a prison-based post and I decided to try working with large groups of people in organisations such as banks under the umbrella approach of team building. With the help of some seed funding from the WCMD, I realised that a brand name would help distance me from the services I was trying to sell. By disassociating myself in this way, I was able to talk about my business, 'Musicatwork', as a separate object, and something that I was part of but that was also bigger and different from 'just me'. Having Musicatwork felt like a protective shield; I could enjoy its successes, and I was protected from its failures, to an extent.

Musicatwork built up, little by little, into a small team of up to eight therapists between 2007 and 2013. As a sole trader, all the risk and responsibility was on my shoulders, but I also had all the freedom to set up and create work in the way that I wanted. As a sole trader, there were minimal legal responsibilities, and accounting was based on an annual three-line financial submission. At the start, my vision for Musicatwork was to provide great music therapy in a range of settings as a small agency. I found the work and then asked good therapists to do it, taking a small commission to cover my time and admin costs. It was very much a one-man band set-up in terms of its day-to-day running and my willingness to find people to work together with, who shared the excitement and the vision.

With hindsight, my inexperience at knowing how to grow a business from start-up to small/medium enterprise (SME) was the limiting factor. Towards the end of 2009, my own clinical work started to burn me out; four days a week working with high-intensity teenagers on the autistic spectrum became too much. I wondered how I could continue to create more music therapy in the world, which completely inspired me, as well as avoid becoming burnt out and over-stressed with the clinical work.

In my personal life at this time, my wife and I were trying, and trying, for a baby. Families were therefore very much in the air, and coupled with my ponderings of where to head in my career, I recalled hearing about a really special parent–child programme in 2005 at the World Congress in Brisbane, Australia. In conversations with Wendy, my wife, whose background was in financial services, we started to imagine the possibility of bringing such programmes to the UK, and building a business that balanced clinical excellence with financial sustainability. Wendy's robust optimistic perspective on the capacity for growth in the therapies marketplace coupled with my memory of a uniquely well-packaged and clinically effective approach, gave me the confidence to act.

Sitting in my home office during a cold December, the Sing&Grow programme (SnG) was only a vague memory from a great conference. I just had a sense, much like we sometimes feel in a therapy session, that we need to say something or play something to match a mood or express a hidden idea; that SnG would be a good thing in the UK. It had been running in Australia since 2001, and was nationally funded from 2005. When I sent the shortest of emails to its then national director, Toni Day, I found an open and interested group of colleagues willing to start a discussion about working with me to bring SnG to the UK.

My email said, 'I'm Dan Thomas, a music therapist in the UK. I really like the sound of Sing&Grow and think it would be great in the UK. There's obviously lots of things that we would need to agree and discuss for this to happen, but are you interested in starting a conversation to make this happen?' Toni responded a few days later positively and there began a partnership that was as much based on personal friendships developing as it was on the success of SnG in the UK. What I had liked about SnG from internet research was its robust evidence base (and an evaluation tool), which was presented in a way that families and commissioners could easily relate to. These three elements meant that it was easy to sell. However, the question of 'Will people pay for it?' became less certain over time, due to factors outside of our control, but predictable nonetheless.

At that time, we didn't fully see or understand how the structure of our business could affect how we were able to operate it, and therefore set up a community interest company (CIC) called 'Sing & Grow UK' in 2010. Through this organisation we could apply for grants, sell the programme directly to commissioners and start to create a brand. SnG had a lovely, friendly identity: bright colours, great information, and focused entirely on early years. Whilst this was one of its strengths, with hindsight, it was also a weakness because we weren't able to diversify and grow into other areas and build on the contacts we had and our good reputation in the early years sector. We were putting a lot of effort into establishing Sing & Grow UK as an organisation without realising that we couldn't expand under that brand; for example Sing & Grow UK could never offer services to adults in mental health settings.

The early years market, in the UK and in many other countries, is vastly underfunded. Nurseries and local councils struggle to fund additional services for those families most in need of help, even with initiatives such as SureStart. Despite facilitating over 100 SnG programmes across the UK, and achieving 'programme recognition' from the Centre for Excellence and Outcomes in Children and Young People's Services (C4EO), SnG in the UK was not sustainable. SnG managed to do the excellent work it achieved because of two factors: the team of experienced and committed music therapists who were at the heart of SnG's clinical effectiveness, and the many hours of pro bono work from the leadership team including our regional coordinators. Pro bono work is often part of setting up new businesses but it doesn't put food on the table, and SnG struggled to become financially sustainable.

The experience of running SnG in the UK was valuable, as I learnt how to inspire and lead a bigger group of therapists and work within a small office-based team of four. However, we came to see that by relying on uncertain grant-based funding streams, we didn't have any financial ability or certainty to invest, grow or scale up our operations. SnG had an evidence base to show it worked, it was packaged in a way that made it easy to talk about and sell to SureStart and other children's centres, but early years commissioners lacked the financial resources to buy it, despite 75 per cent of its cost being offset by the grants that we had been awarded.

Start off with an 'exit strategy'

In 2013, commissions to Musicatwork and Sing & Grow UK started to shrink. The senior leadership team agreed with me that we should start afresh and combine Musicatwork and Sing & Grow UK into a new organisation, Chroma. We took the opportunity to expand our 'offer' to include art therapy, dramatherapy and a range of assessment tools such as APCI (Jacobsen 2013) and MATADOC (Magee *et al.* 2012). I was very clear that we needed to think differently about how we did what we did. I asked for advice from a successful record producer friend, phrasing my question in a simple and unedited way: 'Paul, how do I get my small business to grow into a large business like yours?' His answer was a shock: 'What's your exit strategy?' I had nothing to say. I actually didn't understand the question. I replied, 'Exit strategy? I'm trying to start something, not end it.'

There was something therapeutically resonant in his question – to understand the beginning we often have to think about the ending. In this way the start and the end are connected, and the resonance is about the whole of the work being 'seen' in the first session. Talking to Paul further, it was clear that the exit strategy for Chroma could be managed in two distinct ways. The first exit strategy means the people running it work hard and derive their income from it, but once they retire or close the business that is the end of it – their business stops existing. The owners don't need to focus on adding value in terms of making the business something that someone else would want to buy.

The other type of exit strategy is that the owners hope to sell it on. Decisions are made that allow the business to easily scale up its operations, to enable new revenue streams to be easily added, and company structures put in place which create adaptability and flexibility for any new owners. Relationships may also be built early on in the life of the business which seek to identify potential buyers. In established sectors of the economy such as manufacturing or insurance this is commonplace. However, within the arts therapies marketplace, there is no precedent for businesses such as Chroma being sold/bought, and no guarantee that a buyer would adhere to the high ethical and quality standards that Chroma sets for itself.

Why Chroma?

The name Chroma was chosen with three ideas in mind, which are central to how my colleagues and I see our work going forward. We wanted our business name to:

- not describe what we do (Apple *became* a computer firm; we wanted to Chroma to have the capacity to grow and evolve too)

- be from the world of the arts (Chroma is a fine-art term)

- have something to do with a process or change (Chroma relates to prisms and colour).

The wish to grow, expand and operate Chroma on a day-to-day basis, first and foremost as a clinically excellent, financially sustainable and profitable organisation, is central to how we can support and work with our clients. Businesses only run out of money once before they go bankrupt, and a bankrupt business is no use to a family in need of support, or an adult recovering from a stroke. Our senior leadership team has four therapists and two non-therapists on it; our board of directors is made up of two therapists and one accountant – in this way we hope to ensure that our primary focus always remains clinical excellence, although it is supported by a robust understanding of the financial realities of running a business.

Getting serious

As a music therapist with no formal business training, I am always learning about how to do things more effectively, more efficiently and more seamlessly. My overriding life script of 'be independent' that has driven me thus far remains helpful to a point. However, it is only as I have learnt to collaborate and build a team of people with expertise in required areas (finance, administration, strategy, clinical governance) and by developing partnerships with researchers, supervisors and other professionals, that Chroma has managed to grow. What is valuable in Chroma is our team of therapists, and the good reputation Chroma has is all down to their work, which is supported by the senior leadership team's relentless focus on clinical excellence alongside financial sustainability.

Within the context of ongoing learning, it will continue to be useful to take ideas and processes from other sectors and use them within Chroma. There may be more similarities than differences between an arts therapies business and a financial services business for example, when you take away any moral, political or social judgements on the essential worthiness of either organisation. For example, both are providing a service as opposed to a manufactured product; both rely on transactions of money and service provision through the prism of a relationship (client–therapist or independent financial advisor–customer); and in both, the quality of communication, transparency and reliability are critical to the longevity and trustworthiness of the relationship.

In 2014, Chroma started to work with a marketing company who contacted more than 1000 schools on our behalf, starting a series of conversations with head teachers and special needs coordinators.

We were talking to them about a range of social, emotional and educational support their students required, and exploring whether arts therapy services could work alongside teachers and educators. Using a marketing company to do this initial work would be seen as very commonplace within other business sectors, but within the arts therapies it was considered new, and maybe controversial. Developing a trusting relationship with the marketing company gave us confidence in their ability to communicate successfully and ethically about the arts therapies. We did everything we could to ensure they communicated to potential commissioners and organisational users of arts therapies in a way that was consistent with the core approach of Chroma, which is collaboration.

As an arts therapist, my passion is to increase access to great-quality arts therapy in the world; to help clients, colleagues and commissioners in 'realising potential through creativity' – the Chroma strapline. Becoming serious about moving towards this aim meant imagining Chroma might one day want to run a hospital, or a group of schools. Being called Chroma, as opposed to 'UK Arts Therapies Ltd', for example, means that we are open to those possibilities, however distant or remote they may seem to be.

Next steps

Chroma's core approach is collaborative. We recognise that it is through relationships and face-to-face conversations that new possibilities are brought from imagination to reality. As we have grown over the past few years, the roles and responsibilities of members of the senior leadership team (SLT) have evolved in definition and clarity. This has allowed the management of clinical services to become more effective, whilst allowing those members of the SLT who focus on process and strategy to use their previous experience of working in other sectors (financial planning, insurance, sales) to enable Chroma to grow and expand into new clinical areas. Continually balancing clinical excellence alongside financial sustainability is a challenge but one that is to the ultimate benefit of the clients, patients, children and families that our therapists work with.

As Chroma has grown, and the SLT responsibilities have developed, my role as Managing Director (MD) has also changed.

In 2005 when I started Musicatwork, I was doing everything. Now, as we enter our fourth year as Chroma, but my twelfth year of running a therapy business, what is now required of the MD role allows me to return to my love of building relationships with people (commissioners and therapists primarily) and my passion for finding new clinically effective approaches through which people feel able to access therapy, with my strongly held ethical beliefs about how Chroma should operate in the world. By acknowledging the importance of independence and resilience, and then learning to trust others and work collaboratively, I hope we can move forward and continue what we have started to build.

As I speak to commissioners, I am inspired to hear them describe themselves as passionate advocates of the services they seek to provide. In this way, their work and the work of our art, drama and music therapists feels very linked and closely connected. I've always held a view that great therapy and great business share a common core which is a human-to-human relationship. Regardless of the external influences (diagnoses, capacity, funding, setting or political frameworks), it is the face-to-face conversations that therapists and people involved in the commissioning and delivery of services have that make a difference. We all have to be brave enough to take advantage of those moments, in therapy or in business, when we need to act or react in a compassionate, creative and expansive way, despite our fears. In setting up and running therapy businesses, accepting our role as pioneers (for better or worse) ultimately allows clients to access therapy in settings, locations and through modalities that are meaningful to them. I love having more arts therapies in the world, and it is this simple objective that inspires me each morning and motivates me to share my passion with clients, colleagues and commissioners.

Go and do it!

Exercise 1: Scoping out potential partners

Spend some time to think about which other professionals, outside of the therapy world, you could work with to bring expertise in the non-therapy areas of your business. This might include marketing, finance, and so on.

Exercise 2: Dream, plan, act

Spend some time imagining your business in five years' time – what would it look like, what would you be doing? Use this opportunity to think BIG. Make sure the BIG is something that inspires you. Then write down some initial actions or steps you could take now which move you in that direction.

References

Jacobsen, S.L. (2013). *Clinical application of Assessment of Parenting Competencies (APC)*. Abstract from the 9th European Music Therapy Congress, Oslo, 7–10 August, 2016.

Magee, W. L., Siegert, R. J., Daveson, B. A., Lenton-Smith, G. and Taylor, S.M. (2013). Music therapy assessment tool for awareness in disorders of consciousness (MATADOC): Standardisation of the principal subscale to assess awareness in patients with disorders of consciousness. *Neuropscyhological Rehabilitation: An International Journal.* doi: 10.1080/09602011.2013.844174.

CHAPTER 11

Case Study: Striking a Balance
Music Therapist vs. Businessman in Hong Kong
Kingman Chung

Introduction

Music therapy services started in Hong Kong in the 1980s. The services mainly targeted children with diagnoses such as autistic spectrum disorder (ASD) or attention deficit hyperactivity disorder (ADHD). Music therapy services later extended to geriatric and medical populations. At present Hong Kong music therapists work with a range of clients in a variety of clinical settings including special schools, hospitals and mental health clinics. However, funding for these positions remains challenging and recognition for this profession is severely lacking.

Currently, there are 42 internationally qualified music therapists in Hong Kong (Hong Kong Music Therapy Association 2016). This makes for a vibrant international scene, with music therapists having trained in many countries and being registered to overseas bodies such as the Australian Music Therapy Association, American Music Therapy Association, the British Association for Music Therapy, and Canadian Association for Music Therapy. However, with the lack of a local training facility and no Hong Kong registering body for music therapists, we lack a united front to address funding, policy and public awareness issues as a profession. This means most Hong Kong music therapists are working on their own. Many are doing this as freelance service providers who also work in other areas such as music education. There are also private music therapy centres providing music therapy to individual clients as well as schools and non-profit organisations.

Growing music therapy awareness and practice in Hong Kong

Public awareness of music therapy, due to an increased number of music therapists, music therapy jobs and media coverage, has led to greater interest in the profession. While this is very exciting, there is still a severe lack of understanding of what music therapy actually is, what we do and who we work with. This situation has not improved much since 2012 when I was a fresh graduate from Brisbane, Australia, eager to start my music therapy career in Hong Kong. I was passionate and hopeful about bringing my knowledge and clinical experience back to my home country. It wasn't long before I landed my first job providing a music therapy service to students with ADHD in a mainstream school.

My early experience as a clinician

This first job was referred by an acquaintance, and aimed to improve the attention span of ten students via hourly group music therapy sessions over eight weeks. It was an invaluable experience for me both clinically and as a start-up businessman. Before the programme started, I had no direct communication with the school, nor was I given any background information on any of the clients involved. The organisation told me that I was free to use any form of music therapy intervention in the work. However, I had to use a workbook created by them for assessing attention span. The content of this workbook was not music therapy-related at all. At the same time, the school was not expecting the programme to be a music therapy programme. They expected their students to have visible and significant improvements in their attention span through the help of the workbook. They did not know what music therapy was about or what music therapy could offer. There was an obvious miscommunication between the organisation, the school and myself. Also, I was not given the opportunity to explain my work. As a result, there was a serious misfit between the school's expectation and the service I delivered. Eventually, I became so frustrated that I stopped working with this organisation after the programme ended. After I experienced similar situations with other organisations, I began to think about the possibility of setting up my own music therapy centre.

Rationale for setting up the company

In the short time that I worked for different centres, I felt a lack of support and feedback on the quality of my work. I also realised that in most situations the clients have limited information on music therapy. The clientele of music therapy at that time was very narrow, almost exclusively for children with special needs, or elderly adults. There were clear gaps between the market and the way which music therapy could be delivered. With these ideas in mind, I began setting up my own music therapy centre with the support of a sponsor who shared the same belief in the power of music as me. This sponsor was interested in assisting me to set up the company because he once suffered from anxiety and emotional issues and had to see a psychiatrist. He was subsequently prescribed medication from which he suffered major side-effects such as low motivation and flat affect. The initial struggles I faced as a new music therapist in Hong Kong actually strengthened my belief in music and boosted my passion for promoting and educating the public about the benefits of music therapy. After the sponsor knew what a music therapy service could bring to people with mental health issues (decreased medication, fewer side-effects, increased motivation and engagement, etc.), he suggested that I set up a company to realise my passion and beliefs and said that he would provide financial assistance as his form of support.

International Music Therapy Centre (IMTC)
'Bringing healing through music'

IMTC was established in 2014 to bring about healing through music. IMTC is my business, and is run as a limited company with sponsor support. IMTC began as a small company to meet gaps in the market that I perceived and have outlined above. It has grown to provide music therapy and other psychological services to a wide range of clients via individual and group therapy, psychological support and public education through a team of 14 staff members including music therapists, clinical psychologists, marketing consultants and administration staff. In early 2017, IMTC became the first social enterprise in Hong Kong dedicated to the promotion of music therapy recognised by the Hong Kong Council of Social Service.

At IMTC, our vision is to ensure music therapy becomes an integral and well-accepted form of therapy for people with assessed needs. Our missions are to promote different approaches of music therapy, and to educate the public about the benefits that music can bring to our well-being.

Our missions and vision are based on our core values, which are:

- Passion
  Client-oriented with a strong belief in music: Our colleagues and music therapists strongly believe in the therapeutic benefits that music can bring to the self and to the wider community. Through a client-oriented approach, our team aims to incorporate the individual's strengths to address their needs.

- Creativity
  Fun, motivating and able to think out of the box: Our team is highly flexible in running fun and motivating therapeutic sessions that aim to increase engagement of the client with others, and maximise the therapeutic outcome within the music.

- Evidence-based
  Scientific and professional: Music as a therapeutic medium has gained much attention in the world of research in recent years. We believe that it is vital to keep up to date with the latest music therapy research in order to better inform our therapy work with clients. It is our responsibility to provide ethical and professional therapy services to all our clients.

- Teamwork
  Multi-approaches and supports: We believe that different music therapy approaches are better suited for different settings. Each therapist has their individual unique strength, passion and expertise. Therefore, in the process of developing the market, each therapist is encouraged to develop their own career pathway. When a new therapist starts their work at our centre, we have a discussion about their area of passion, personal musical skills, personal therapeutic style and approach, as well as past experience. We also have a

conversation about the career path that they have in mind. IMTC aims to collaborate, explore and create relevant opportunities for them. If and when the therapist needs more time and experiences to better understand what career path is suitable, IMTC is also open to providing various different opportunities to assist in this process.

Present marketing directions: explorations and innovations

Currently, music therapy work is mostly steered towards a traditional top-down approach. I believe that in order to set up long-term sustainable music therapy programmes, we need to comprehend the real needs of the client/community to determine where music can play a therapeutic role across different settings. Often when we set up a new music therapy programme, there are multiple factors that need to be considered and compromised on. I present some of these considerations in the following case examples.

Cancer choir in a hospital

Cancer patients often face feelings of anxiety and depression. A cancer diagnosis may also lower their self-esteem, negatively affect their relationship with their family and lead to social isolation (Wormit *et al.* 2012). Research shows that music therapy (MT) intervention can assist oncology patients in many ways, including significantly improving quality of life, decreasing stress related to the oncology treatment, alleviating pain, and minimising the side-effects from treatment (Bradt *et al.* 2011; Mahon & Mahon 2011). Music therapy delivered through choir settings has also led to decreased feelings of depression amongst participants (Petchkovsky *et al.* 2013).

Based on the literature and research in cancer care, I set up a three-year music therapy programme at a cancer day centre located in a hospital. It involved a choir for people with cancer and/or their carers and small-group programmes as well as individual music therapy services. The programme was based on expectations from three parties:

- the funding body – looking for innovative programmes that could incorporate a larger group of people and have the potential to receive wider media coverage to increase public awareness of well-being

- the non-governmental organisation (NGO) – looking for therapeutic services that could serve their clients to improve quality of life

- the music therapist – looking for an opportunity to extend the services offered in Hong Kong.

This programme is currently ongoing. In the choir, a typical therapy session begins with a music and muscle relaxation exercise that involves live piano music and different types of muscle relaxation exercises, followed by vocal warm-up exercises. Then there will be some vocal improvisation exercises, after which there will be song practice. The session consistently ends with the Chinese song called 'Friends' that was chosen by the clients. In addition to the weekly therapy session, the choir often performs at various settings including hospitals, community centres and public events. These performances aim to:

- increase self-esteem

- provide opportunities for clients to create a sense of achievement

- increase public awareness of this choir and music therapy services for the cancer population.

Stroke choir in a rehabilitation centre

One year after the cancer choir had started, I began to ponder the possibility of starting a stroke choir in Hong Kong. During my years of study in Australia, I saw a performance by the Stroke a Chord choir, aimed at giving a voice to people with Broca's aphasia after a stroke. Through my work connections, I realised that the rehabilitation services available to people suffering from strokes in Hong Kong were quite limited. Research has shown that choir singing for people who have experienced a stroke can lead to significant improvements in quality-of-life measures for the participants (Tamplin *et al.* 2013). Therefore, I began to plan the creation of the first stroke choir in Hong Kong by looking for interested organisations. Initially, many organisations turned down the proposal for a variety of reasons, such as funding, or that they were simply not looking for this type of service. After much perseverance, I finally got in touch with an organisation that supported and believed in this idea. We worked on funding applications and after many initial failed attempts, we secured three-year funding to start this choir.

This programme is currently also ongoing. The structure of each therapy session is similar to that of the cancer choir, with a heavier emphasis on singing familiar songs to facilitate speech. Most clients in this choir are diagnosed with Broca's aphasia. In addition to speech rehabilitation, other goals include increasing self-esteem and social supports to members of the choir.

From the above case examples, I hope you can see that in order to create new programmes, we can't simply think or communicate from a music therapist's perspective. We need to combine our knowledge and expectation to create new programmes alongside realistic expectations as a negotiator. On the one hand, as a music therapist I believe in the therapeutic effects that music can bring when applied in a systematic and informed manner. On the other, I believe that music has a positive impact on the community at large, and multiple parties in the community have their role to play. Combine the two beliefs and new innovative programmes and opportunities can be created.

Leaving the comfort zone, thinking outside the box

For a centre to be financially sustainable, it is essential that the marketing direction matches the core values of the society and culture where it is located. Hong Kong is one of the world's leading international financial hubs. It is also one of the world's most densely populated metropolises with around 7.2 million people living a very fast pace of life. From my observation, there are two main characteristics in the Hong Kong culture:

- *Time efficiency:* In Hong Kong, most people lead very busy lives, playing multiple roles – fathers, sons, employers, employees, and so on. At the same time, Hong Kong has the highest weekly working hours in the world (Statista 2015). In order to fulfil the expectations of these roles, people have to make sure that everything is handled in a time-efficient manner so that they can meet the seemingly never-ending commitments on their plates.

- *Cost efficiency:* Hong Kong is one of the world's leading economic hubs. This also means that being sensitive to money is one of the most common traits across all organisations. In addition, Hong Kong has a very limited pool of resources for a large population, having one of the world's highest population densities. Hence it is very important to make sure that any project, big or small, is proven to be cost-efficient before it can be accepted.

Due to these two characteristics, people in Hong Kong tend to work in a target-oriented manner. As a result, it is highly likely that people living in Hong Kong face pressure from various aspects of their lives, especially in their workplace. This lifestyle has a great impact on the individual's psychosocial well-being. From a corporation's point of view, this impact may directly affect the employees' work quality and efficiency. Therefore, corporations are generally interested in programmes that address two big needs:

- individual employees' mental well-being

- team dynamic and bonding.

Once we have identified the real needs of the local culture and society, we then think outside the box and design programmes where music can meet the specific needs within that culture. These programmes may not be marketed or run as traditional therapy programmes (one-off session, full-day workshop), but are tailor-made to suit each corporation.

In addition, there is a certain stigma attached to the word 'therapy' in the Hong Kong culture. When dealing with corporations, I think it is important to reiterate that our knowledge and experience as music therapists are vital to running a good programme. However, it may be more feasible to present the programme as a non-therapy programme to increase their engagement in what is being offered within this cultural context.

Case example: 'impossible to possible' – a collaboration with an insurance company

IMTC collaborated with an insurance company for a one-time project that aimed to improve team bonding and increase motivation for better work performance. The programme involved 200 employees at one of the world's biggest insurance companies. It involved a one-hour-fifteen-minute music experience in which a small group of participants learnt to sing the song 'Gangnam Style' and the rest learnt to play the ukulele to accompany the singers. At the end of this experience, the two groups came together to perform for everyone. Through this process, they got to experience the process of working together towards a common goal through a fun and seemingly impossible process (learning to play the ukulele in 45 minutes?!) to create a memorable outcome. On top of this, the company also wished to use this programme as an interesting way to inform their employees that they would be rewarded with a trip to Korea if they met a certain level of work performance.

This was a very exciting initial collaboration between IMTC and a corporate company. We continue to promote other programmes that focus on improving the well-being of employees but also continue to get mixed feedback. It appears that despite strong links between employees' well-being and work performance (Taris & Schaufeli 2015), this approach has not become a common trend in employee benefits across Hong Kong corporations at the moment.

The current scene at IMTC: our services

Music as a medium is widely accessible, and deeply ingrained in our everyday lives. Within the Hong Kong society, music therapists can offer their services to people with differing background and needs. At IMTC, we have two forms of services:

- Music therapy services:
  - » To provide music therapy sessions and/ or workshops to those in need:
    - – individual clients and their family (paediatric to geriatric)

- – schools (mainstream and special school)
- – NGOs
- – hospitals.
  - » To provide music therapy programmes for employees:
    - – NGOs
    - – hospitals
    - – corporations.
- Community music and music therapy services:
  - » To provide music therapy and music-related services to the community in order to enhance the community social responsibility.
  - » To increase cooperation with musicians and other people in the music industry.

Challenge: therapist vs. businessman

One of the biggest challenges and dilemmas I have faced so far is striking a balance between being a good therapist and being a successful businessman. As a therapist, I deeply value empathy and compassion. It is my instinctive reaction to put myself in my clients' shoes, trying my very best to understand their situations and difficulties. I often find it difficult to let go of any opportunity to help people through music. However, as a businessman, I understand the importance of being realistic in running the centre. When potential clients express their inability to pay for the music therapy services, tough decisions have to be made – should I provide free services or turn them away? Because this situation keeps arising, I began to think of ways to create a win-win situation.

Solutions

- Refer the potential clients to NGOs.
  Although it is difficult for IMTC to apply for funding as it is a limited company, we actively cooperate with many

NGOs in writing proposals to secure funding to support music therapy programmes. When a client expresses financial difficulties, we often refer them to NGOs in their local area.

- Use a sliding scale fee structure for people experiencing financial difficulties.

   Music therapy services are still not widely available across Hong Kong to meet the needs of many. Therefore, we came up with a separate price range for therapy services delivered by our centre. Should the clients be able to prove their lack of finances (by registered social workers), they would be eligible for a special price range.

- Provide regular community services.

   IMTC firmly believes in having, and acting to support, community social responsibility. We believe we have an important part to play in contributing to public health and well-being through music across Hong Kong. We hold free workshops and talks to the community through NGOs or public events on a regular basis.

Challenge: marketing of self vs. the team

When I began IMTC I prioritised marketing the company and its vision, mission and value. I tried to avoid marketing myself as an individual therapist as I believe that a therapist should keep their professional boundaries with clients. Also, I felt that music therapy should not be represented by any individual alone, for the best therapy work is achieved through team effort.

Solution

The reality for me, and probably many other business owners, is this: it is hard to separate oneself from the centre because the centre reflects and realises one's own vision – the centre is me. The public media also tend to focus on an individual rather than a centre. As a result, I began to accept my role as a spokesperson and advocate for my company as well as our team members.

Personal reflections
Setting goals and objectives in your business

As music therapists, we always set up goals and objectives after assessing our clients' needs. And we all know that goal-setting is very important. It is similar in business. Goal-setting is very important because it can help you to organise your time and resources so that you can make more opportunities to achieve your goals. It is also an excellent way to turn your idea into an action.

I define and measure goals as follows:

- goals: what you want to achieve in the future

- sub-goals: what you need to do to realise your goals

- objectives: what the specific actions are that can accomplish your sub-goals.

Examples from IMTC

Goal:

- Within five years, to form a team of music therapists with expertise in children with autism spectrum disorder.

Sub-goals:

- Within one year, we will have at least five music therapists who would like to commit to the team.

- The team will present at the Autism Spectrum Disorders Symposium within two years.

- The team will publish articles in *Children and Health Magazine* within 18 months.

Objectives:

- Every two weeks, I will look for suitable therapists and share my ideas with them.

- Every month, we will have a two-hour meeting to prepare the presentation for the Autism Spectrum Disorders Symposium.

- We will write an article about music therapy and ASD and then pitch it to the media on a monthly basis.

Striking a balance

Since the establishment of IMTC, the biggest lesson I have learnt is how hard it can be to strike a balance between your aspirations and reality. Once you have set a goal, it is important to keep in mind the cultural context so that your goal is attainable. When I faced challenges in designing new programmes, I formulated a series of steps that I found useful:

- Is there a need for services?

- Does it call to our areas of passion?

- Is it possible to execute within the current economic situation?

- Are there ways to make it sustainable?

I found this model a good combination of my beliefs as a therapist and also my role as a businessman. I do not believe that a therapist and businessman are in constant conflict. There are ways in which one can inform the other to achieve a more ideal outcome. As both a businessman and a therapist, I often remind myself to never stop reflecting on my therapy work and also the business' directions. Lastly, it is important to have frequent discussions with your teammates, and develop strong team bonding and trust so that you develop the music therapy industry in a shared direction.

Holding on to your beliefs

Managing a business whilst being a therapist is no easy feat. In the process of trying to come to different compromises and meeting different expectations, I have struggled on many occasions with the ways in which music therapy is being communicated or delivered in different settings. Over time, I began to realise the importance of holding onto your own core beliefs about your profession and knowing when to say 'no', even when this means compromising the creation of a new programme/service. In addition, seeking advice from other therapists, especially those in your team, can be very valuable. One can often paint a clearer and more complete picture with input from various perspectives, whereas this process can be all but impossible to do by yourself.

Building recognition of the profession

One of the biggest challenges in doing marketing work at IMTC is the lack of recognition of the music therapy profession in Hong Kong. In addition to this, I feel the lack of local research also contributes greatly to this phenomenon. Without local research, it will be a very long and hard journey to gain government recognition for music therapy services. This means that the problem of funding will be long term, which may not be helpful to the development of a music therapy service in Hong Kong. Therefore, IMTC is looking to start some pilot research studies in collaboration with our existing programmes. The stroke choir is one example of this. We are currently doing a research paper that investigates the impact of weekly choir practice on speech ability of patients with Broca's aphasia (selected from clients in the stroke choir).

What is success? What is failure?

Everyone has a different idea of what success and failure mean, whether it be in their life, career or family. For me, I am privileged to be able to use the IMTC as a platform on which I can spread and share music therapy services in my home country, supported by a team of colleagues. However, if one day I am no longer able to be supported by a centre, I would not think that I have failed. I believe the size or scale of a business does not equate to the success of my career as a music therapist. I think it is important not to let the idea of running a business overtake my belief and value of being who I am – a music therapist.

Conclusion

Since starting my own centre, I have faced many opportunities as well as challenges, be it in learning how to run a business or my own self-development as a music therapist, all within the cultural context and backdrop of Hong Kong. Reflecting on the past few years, one point stands out amongst the rest: never under- or overestimate the impact of your work. Whether as a music therapist or a businessman, the impact you make, for the clients and/or music therapy scene, may not always be immediate or tangible. However, I believe that as long as you remain client-oriented, keep to your passions and maintain your professionalism, you will create a positive impact no matter how challenging the current situation may be.

Go and do it!

Exercise 1: Thinking big: creating a sustainable programme

Write down three ways you can increase public awareness of music therapy in your local community right now. Then apply these questions to your ideas:

- Is there a need for services?

- Does it call to your areas of passion?

- Is it possible to execute within the current economic situation?

- Are there ways to make it sustainable?

Now compile your answers into four paragraphs which can be the backbone of your plan.

Exercise 2: Understanding your culture

Can you outline three things that are specific to the cultural context of where you live and identify how these impact on the citizens, the way they live and the way they work? How can a music therapy programme tap into this?

Exercise 3: Starting small: Setting up goals and objectives

For your plan above, write one goal, two sub-goals and three objectives that can help you make this a reality. These are the steps you will take to increase the public awareness of music therapy in your local community.

Exercise 4: Strengthen your beliefs

- What is success to you? Can you define it or capture it in one sentence?

- What is failure to you? Can you define it or capture it in one sentence?

- Now can you find a way to take your failure and make it a success by focusing on your core beliefs?

Note: I would like to extend my heartfelt gratitude to Angela Ho (RMT) for her support in writing this chapter. I would also like to say a big thank you to every person who has appeared in my life, without whom I would not be who I am today.

References

Bradt, J., Dileo, C., Grocke, D. and Magill, L. (2011). Music interventions for improving psychological and physical outcomes in cancer patients. *Cochrane Database System Review*, 10, 8.

Hong Kong Music Therapy Association. (2016). *Home Page*. Retrieved from www.musictherapyhk.org/registeredmusictherapisthk on 16 January 2017.

Mahon, E.M. and Mahon, S.M. (2011). A valuable adjunct in the oncology setting. *Clinical Journal of Oncology Nursing*, 15, 4, 353–356.

Petchkovsky, L., Roertson-Gillam, K., Kropotov, Y. and Petchkovsky, M. (2013). Using QEEG parameters (asymmetry, coherence, and P3a novelty response) to track improvement in depression after choir therapy. *Advances in Mental Health*, 11, 3, 257–267.

Statista (2015). *Average working hours per year of workers in selected cities around the world in 2015*. Retrieved from www.statista.com/statistics/275497/working-hours-cities on 1 December 2016.

Tamplin, J., Baker, F., Jones, B., Way, A. and Lee, S. (2013). 'Stroke a chord': The effect of singing in a community choir on mood and social engagement for people living with aphasia following a stroke. *NeuroRehabilitation*, 32, 929–941.

Taris, T.W. and Schaufeli, W.B. (2015). Individual Well-being and Performance at Work: A Conceptual and Theoretical Overview. In M. van Veldhoven and R. Peccei (eds) *Well-being and Performance at Work: The role of context* (pp.24-43). London: Psychology Press.

Van Veldhoven, M. and Peccei, R. (eds) (2015). *Well-Being and Performance at Work: The Role of Context.* Hove: Psychology Press.

Wormit, A., Marth, M., Koeing, J., Hillecke, T. and Bardenheuer, H. (2012). Evaluating a treatment manual for music therapy in adult outpatient oncology care. *Music and Medicine,* 4, 2, 65–73.

About the Authors

Vicky Abad (BAMus, PGDip(MT), Med(Research), PhD candidate, RMT) is a registered music therapist, mother, business owner and researcher. She is the Managing Director of Boppin' Babies, and is proud to still work as a clinician each week with families, while also working as a researcher in the area of music early learning, families and music therapy. Vicky is an internationally regarded speaker and researcher and is currently the President of the Australian Music Therapy Association.

Kingman Chung (MMT, RMT, NM) is a registered music therapist with a special focus on serving cancer and stroke patients. He is the founder of the International Music Therapy Centre (IMTC), the first social enterprise in Hong Kong that dedicates itself to the promotion of music therapy. Kingman starts his chairmanship of the Hong Kong Music Therapy Association in 2017. He has also served as an executive committee member of Making Music Being Well (Hong Kong) since 2012.

Elena Fitzthum (Dr sc. mus.) is a certified music therapist, psycho-therapist and supervisor. She is a lecturer at the University of Music and Performing Arts Vienna, Austria, and at Zurich University of the Arts, Switzerland. Her focus of scientific work is the history of music therapy. She is co-founder and President of the Viennese Institute of Music Therapy (WIM), and Austrian delegate to the European Music Therapy Confederation since 2006, serving as board member from 2013 to 2016. She was also a member of the Local Organising Committee of the 10th European Music Therapy Conference 2016 in Vienna, Austria.

Monika Geretsegger (PhD) is a certified music therapist, a clinical and health psychologist and also has a master's degree in linguistics. She is Senior Researcher at GAMUT – The Grieg Academy Music Therapy Research Centre, Uni Research Health, in Bergen, Norway.

In her clinical work, she specialises in children with autism spectrum disorders and adults with mental health problems. She has been a board member of the Austrian Association of Music Therapists (ÖBM) since 2008, serving as President from 2010 to 2016. She was also a member of the Local Organising Committee of the 10th European Music Therapy Conference 2016 in Vienna, Austria.

Stine Lindahl Jacobsen (PhD) is Assistant Professor and Head of the Music Therapy Programme Aalborg University, Denmark. As the head of the MA programme at Aalborg University, she aims to offer education that will help music therapy students develop competencies of integrity. She has a clinical background and insights into both private and public practices. Her expertise in ethics, marketing and transparency comes from her private practice experience as the owner of a small for-profit company providing music therapy assessment, training and counselling in the context of vulnerable families and child protection.

Petra Kern (PhD, MT-BC, MTA, DMtG) is the owner of Music Therapy Consulting and adjunct Associate Professor at the University of Louisville, USA. A former President of the World Federation of Music Therapy (WFMT), author of over 60 publications, and recipient of several national and international awards, Dr Kern continues to serve as editor-in-chief of *imagine*, is on the Board of Directors of the Certification Board of Music Therapy (CBMT) and sits on various committees while being an active international speaker and guest lecturer. She likes to see her students become well equipped with knowledge, skills and resources to face the demands of a business-driven global world.

Alison Ledger (PhD) completed her undergraduate and Masters studies in music therapy at the University of Queensland, Australia. After several years of working as a music therapist in health and educational settings, it struck her that business development aspects were often the most difficult parts of the job. She therefore decided to study music therapists' experiences of service development for her PhD, completed at the University of Limerick, Ireland, in 2010. Since then, Alison has taught music therapy students in Australia, Ireland, Norway and the U.S., been a pioneer in developing music therapy research methods, and now lectures and supervises research at the Leeds Institute of Medical Education, UK.

Thomas Stegemann (Univ.-Prof. Dr. med. Dr. sc. mus.) is a child and adolescent psychiatrist, licensed music therapist, and family therapist. He also completed studies in guitar (GIT, Los Angeles), and in business administration in healthcare. Since 2011 he has served as Professor of Music Therapy and Head of the Department of Music Therapy at the University of Music and Performing Arts Vienna, Austria, where he is also Deputy Dean of the Department of Scientific Studies. He is co-founder and member of ÖMAK (Austrian Music Therapy Education Conference) and was also a member of the Local Organising Committee and Co-Head of the Scientific Committee of the 10th European Music Therapy Conference 2016 in Vienna, Austria.

Daniel Thomas (BA Hons, PGDip(MT)) qualified as a music therapist in 2002. His clinical work has focused on children and families, especially supporting attachment, bonding and resilience. Daniel has worked in prisons, mental health settings and in special and mainstream schools with children on the Autistic Spectrum. Since 2013, he has been the Managing Director of Chroma, and has a passion for developing business models that allow high quality therapy services to be delivered at scale.

Elaine Matthews Venter is a registered arts therapist in private practice, in Auckland, New Zealand. She works with adults, children and groups. Prior to undertaking the arts therapy qualification, Elaine lectured in art history at the University of Fort Hare, and the Nelson Mandela Metropolitan University in South Africa. She is actively engaged in her own artistic practice and exhibits her work on a regular basis.

Rebecca Zarate (PhD, MT-BC, LCAT, AVPT) is Assistant Professor, music therapy coordinator and doctoral faculty in the division of expressive therapies at Lesley University. Dr Zarate has been a practising music therapist for 16 years, serving a wide range of communities in clinical, educational and leadership roles. Dr Zarate's interests are in the presence and meaning of anxiety and difference in communities, creative arts therapies programme development and training, serving community, shaping policy, and social transformation through artistic enquiry. Dr Zarate is also invested in using her critical improvisation approach with clinical and collective anxiety. She publishes and presents on improvisation, community leadership, community transformation, clinical and collective anxiety. Most recent projects include an awarded faculty research fellowship exploring the impact of critical improvisation methods on community/campus safety and anxiety as a response to increasing violence on college campuses in the US.

Subject Index

Author Index